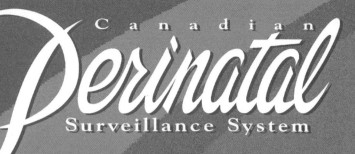

Canadian
Perinatal
Surveillance System

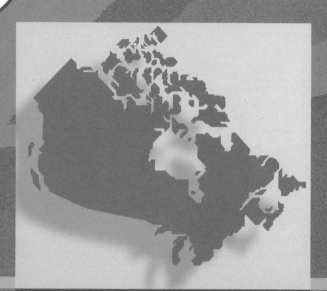

Canadian Perinatal Health Report

2000

Our mission is to help the people of Canada
maintain and improve their health.
Health Canada

Copies of this report are available from:

Reproductive Health Division
Bureau of Reproductive and Child Health
Centre for Healthy Human Development
Population and Public Health Branch
Health Canada
HPB Bldg. #7, A.L. 0701D
Tunney's Pasture
Ottawa, Ontario
K1A 0L2

Telephone: (613) 941-2395
Fax: (613) 941-9927

This publication can also be accessed electronically via the Internet at:
http://www.hc-sc.gc.ca/hpb/lcdc/brch/reprod.html

Également disponible en français sous le titre :
Rapport sur la santé périnatale au Canada, 2000

Suggested citation: Health Canada. Canadian Perinatal Health Report, 2000.
Ottawa: Minister of Public Works and Government Services Canada, 2000.

Published by authority of the Minister of Health

Table of Contents

Section A Determinants of Maternal, Fetal and Infant Health

Section B Maternal, Fetal and Infant Health Outcomes

Table of Contents

List of Figures and Tables

Figures

List of Figures and Tables

List of Figures and Tables

List of Figures and Tables

Tables

Introduction

The *Canadian Perinatal Health Report, 2000* is the first national surveillance report from the Canadian Perinatal Surveillance System (CPSS), and was produced by Health Canada's Bureau of Reproductive and Child Health and the CPSS Steering Committee. Together, the Bureau and the Steering Committee have developed the conceptual framework for the CPSS, identified appropriate perinatal health indicators and their data sources, and undertaken analysis and interpretation of the data. This report and subsequent national surveillance reports (to be released at regular intervals) will be complemented by the ongoing publication of fact sheets and peer-reviewed scientific papers.

The CPSS has prepared a companion document to this and future surveillance reports: *Perinatal Health Indicators for Canada: A Resource Manual.*[1] This manual, which provides information on the indicators being monitored by the CPSS, is intended as a reference guide for readers of this national surveillance report and for those undertaking perinatal health data collection, analysis, interpretation and response at provincial, territorial or regional levels.

Background

The Bureau of Reproductive and Child Health began the development of the CPSS in 1995, as part of Health Canada's initiative to fill gaps in national public health surveillance. The work of the Canadian Perinatal Regionalization Coalition (now the Canadian Perinatal Programs Coalition) on the development of a national perinatal database was an important foundation for the CPSS. The CPSS collaborates with Statistics Canada, the Canadian Institute for Health Information (CIHI), provincial and territorial governments, health professional organizations, advocacy groups and university-based researchers. Representatives of these groups and several international experts serve on the CPSS Steering Committee and its study groups. The mission, principles and objectives of the CPSS are described elsewhere.[2,3]

CPSS Conceptual Framework

The CPSS considers a health surveillance system to be a core system of ongoing data collection, analysis and interpretation on vital public health issues. The result is information that is used to develop and evaluate interventions, with the aim of reducing health disparities and promoting health.[2] Figure I depicts the cycle of surveillance, adapted from a conceptual framework described by Dr. Brian McCarthy, Centers for Disease Control and Prevention, Atlanta, Georgia.[4]

The CPSS considers a health surveillance system to be a core system of ongoing data collection, analysis and interpretation on vital public health issues. The result is information that is used to develop and evaluate interventions, with the aim of reducing health disparities and promoting health.

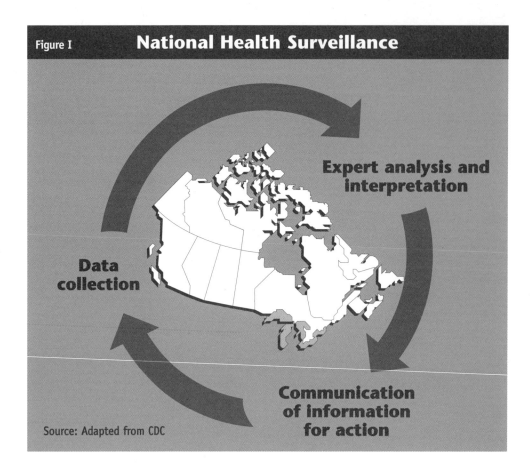

Figure I — **National Health Surveillance**

Data collection

Expert analysis and interpretation

Communication of information for action

Source: Adapted from CDC

Overlying this concept of health surveillance is the concept of the determinants of health: that health status is influenced by a range of factors including, but not limited to, health care.[5] Therefore, it is important to monitor not only health outcomes, but also factors — such as behaviours, physical and social environments, and health services — that may affect those outcomes. Health surveillance aims to contribute to improved health outcomes — that is the end point. However, information on trends and patterns in various risk and protective factors helps to explain patterns of morbidity and mortality, and may point the way to effective interventions and allocation of health resources that will improve outcomes. Monitoring of health determinants and monitoring of health outcomes go hand in hand in health surveillance systems.

CPSS Indicators

A health indicator is "a measurement that, when compared to either a standard or desired level of achievement, provides information regarding a health outcome or important health determinant."[2] The Bureau of Reproductive and Child Health and the CPSS Steering Committee undertook a process to identify the perinatal health indicators that should be monitored by a national perinatal surveillance system.[1] The group considered the importance of the health outcome or determinant, the scientific properties of the indicator, such as its validity in measuring that outcome or determinant, and the feasibility of collecting the data required to construct it. Appendix B contains the set of indicators that resulted from this process. The first 43 indicators listed are ranked according to the Steering Committee's assessment of health importance. Nine additional indicators were added to the list after subsequent consultations.

The principal data sources currently available for national perinatal health surveillance are described in Appendix A and in more detail in *Perinatal Health Indicators for Canada*. Using these available data sources (vital statistics, hospitalization data and national health surveys), the CPSS can report on only a subset of the indicators in Appendix B. The program is supporting efforts to improve existing databases and fill data gaps. This work, accompanied by ongoing developments in information technology and health information systems, will provide more perinatal health data at the national level, so that the number of indicators on which the CPSS can report will increase, as will our ability to understand and explain temporal trends and geographic and other disparities in the indicators.

Outline of the Report

This report contains information on 24 perinatal health indicators, grouped as indicators of health determinants (behaviours and practices and health services) and indicators of outcomes (maternal, fetal and infant health). For each indicator, surveillance results are presented, data limitations discussed and key references listed. Statistics for each indicator consist mainly of temporal trends at the national level and interprovincial/territorial comparisons for the most recent year for which data are available.

Summary

Perinatal health surveillance is a necessary component of managing the health system to improve the health status of pregnant women, mothers and infants in Canada. It is far more than a static database for perinatal health. Rather, it comprises a dynamic, integrated system of data collection, linkage, validation, analysis, interpretation and reporting that permits timely identification of "red flags," tracking of temporal trends and geographic and other disparities, as well as assessment of the effect of changes in clinical practice and public health policy. Perinatal health surveillance provides both a measurement tool (where we have been in the past, where we are at present) and a stimulus to action (where we need to be in the future).

Perinatal health surveillance provides both a measurement tool (where we have been in the past, where we are at present) and a stimulus to action (where we need to be in the future).

Michael S. Kramer, MD
Professor of Epidemiology and
 Biostatistics and Pediatrics
McGill University
Chairperson, CPSS Steering
 Committee

Catherine McCourt, MD, MHA, FRCPC
Director, Bureau of Reproductive and
 Child Health
Centre for Healthy Human Development
Population and Public Health Branch
Health Canada

References

1. Health Canada. *Perinatal Health Indicators for Canada: A Resource Manual.* Ottawa: Minister of Public Works and Government Services Canada, 2000 (Catalogue No. H49-135/2000E).

2. Health Canada. *Canadian Perinatal Surveillance System Progress Report.* Ottawa: Minister of Supply and Services Canada, 1995.

3. Health Canada. *Canadian Perinatal Surveillance System Progress Report 1997-1998.* Ottawa: Minister of Public Works and Government Services Canada, 1999.

4. McCarthy B. The risk approach revisited: A critical review of developing country experience and its use in health planning. In: Liljestrand J, Povey WG (Eds.), *Maternal Health Care in an International Perspective. Proceedings of the XXII Berzelius Symposium, 1991 May 27-29, Stockholm, Sweden.* Sweden: Uppsala University, 1992: 107-24.

5. Federal, Provincial and Territorial Advisory Committee on Population Health. *Strategies for Population Health: Investing in the Health of Canadians.* Ottawa: Minister of Supply and Services Canada, 1994.

Contributors

Authors

Tye Arbuckle, PhD
Susie Dzakpasu, MHSc
Shiliang Liu, MB, PhD
Jocelyn Rouleau
I.D. Rusen, MD, MSc, FRCPC
Linda Turner, PhD
Shi Wu Wen, MB, PhD

Editors

Susie Dzakpasu, MHSc
K.S. Joseph, MD, PhD
I.D. Rusen, MD, MSc, FRCPC

Research Assistants

Jennifer Haughton
Fay McLaughlin, RN, BScN

Administrative Support

Ernesto Delgado

Canadian Perinatal Surveillance System Steering Committee Members (2000)

Chairperson

Michael Kramer, MD
Departments of Pediatrics and
  Epidemiology and Biostatistics
McGill University
Montréal, Québec

Representatives

Alexander Allen, MD, FRCPC
Canadian Perinatal Programs
  Coalition
Halifax, Nova Scotia

Madeline Boscoe, RN
Women's Health Network
Winnipeg, Manitoba

Christine Fitzgerald
Canadian Institute for Health
  Information
Ottawa, Ontario

Maureen Heaman, RN, MN, PhD(c)
Association of Women's Health,
  Obstetric and Neonatal Nurses
Canadian Nurses Association
Winnipeg, Manitoba

Pearl Herbert, BN, BEd, MSc
Canadian Confederation of
 Midwives
St. John's, Newfoundland

Sue Hodges, RN, BScN
Canadian Institute of Child Health
Ottawa, Ontario

Vania Jimenez, MDCM, CCFP, FCFP
College of Family Physicians of
 Canada
Montréal, Québec

Robert Liston, MB, ChB, FRCSC,
 FRCOG
Society of Obstetricians and
 Gynaecologists of Canada
Vancouver, British Columbia

Ken Milne, MD, FSOGC, FRCSC
Society of Obstetricians and
 Gynaecologists of Canada
Ottawa, Ontario

Patricia Niday, EdD
Canadian Perinatal Programs
 Coalition
Ottawa, Ontario

Reg Sauve, MD, MPH, FRCPC
Canadian Paediatric Society
Calgary, Alberta

Marianne Stewart, BScN, MHSA
Canadian Public Health Association
Edmonton, Alberta

Individual Experts

Beverley Chalmers, PhD
The Centre for Research in Women's
 Health
University of Toronto
Toronto, Ontario

K.S. Joseph, MD, PhD
Departments of Obstetrics and
 Gynecology and Pediatrics
Dalhousie University
Halifax, Nova Scotia

Judith Lumley, MB, PhD
Centre for the Study of Mothers'
 and Children's Health
La Trobe University
Carlton, Victoria, Australia

Sylvie Marcoux, MD, PhD
Associate Dean, Research
Université Laval
Québec, Québec

Brian McCarthy, MD
Centers for Disease Control and
 Prevention
Atlanta, Georgia, U.S.A.

Arne Ohlsson, MD, MSc, FRCPC
Departments of Paediatrics,
 Obstetrics and Gynaecology,
 Public Health Sciences
University of Toronto
Toronto, Ontario

Federal Government Representatives

Alexa Brewer, MBA, BScN
First Nations and Inuit Health
 Branch
Health Canada
Ottawa, Ontario

Gary Catlin
Health Statistics Division
Statistics Canada
Ottawa, Ontario

Martha Fair
Occupational and Environmental
 Health Research Section
Statistics Canada
Ottawa, Ontario

Carolyn Harrison
Child, Youth and Family Health Section
Health Canada
Ottawa, Ontario

The State of Perinatal Health in Canada

This report on perinatal health in Canada represents an important initiative of the Canadian Perinatal Surveillance System (CPSS). Available information on determinants and outcomes related to fetal, infant and maternal health has been compiled from various sources and provides a broad description of the state of perinatal health in Canada. The focus has been on documenting the magnitude of specific indicators of perinatal health and describing temporal trends and interprovincial/territorial differences in indicator values. This overview briefly summarizes specific topics of contemporary concern in perinatal health and highlights areas requiring attention from a public health, health care or surveillance standpoint.

Overview of Perinatal Health in Canada

Infant Mortality

It appears to be the best of times for perinatal health in Canada, at least when assessed in terms of infant mortality. Infant mortality rates in Canada have declined substantially over the last several decades and are among the lowest in the world. Perhaps as noteworthy is the reduction in regional disparities in infant mortality rates (Figure 1). The magnitude of the reduction in infant mortality since the early 1960s (i.e., before the introduction of national medical insurance) has been higher in provinces and territories where the infant mortality rate was the highest in the early 1960s.[1] For example, the Northwest Territories and the Yukon, which had the highest rates of infant mortality four decades ago (92.9 and 42.0 per 1,000 live births in 1961-1965, respectively) achieved the largest reductions in infant mortality by 1991-1995 (82% and 86% reduction, respectively). This is in contrast to the substantial but relatively smaller reductions in infant mortality (between 68% and 81%) that occurred elsewhere in Canada.[1]

Since enactment of the *Medicare Act* in 1968, the Canadian experience contrasts with the international situation where relative differences between nations have increased; countries with low rates of infant mortality have posted much larger declines than those with higher rates.[1] Although some industrialized countries have slightly lower rates than Canada, the ranking of countries based on small differences in infant mortality is compromised because birth registration practices are not standardized, especially for live births near the borderline of viability.[2,3]

Between 1990 and 1995, Canadian infant mortality rates fluctuated between 6.1 and 6.8 per 1,000 live births (see chapter 4). The crude infant mortality rate in 1993 (6.3 per 1,000 live births) exceeded the infant mortality rate of the previous year (6.1 per 1,000 live births) for the first time in several decades. This led to reports about the dire state of perinatal health in Canada.[4] Diverse factors

It appears to be the best of times for perinatal health in Canada, at least when assessed in terms of infant mortality. Infant mortality rates in Canada have declined substantially over the last several decades and are among the lowest in the world.

FIGURE 1 **Temporal trends in infant mortality rates in provinces/territories,** *Canada, 1961-1965 to 1991-1995*

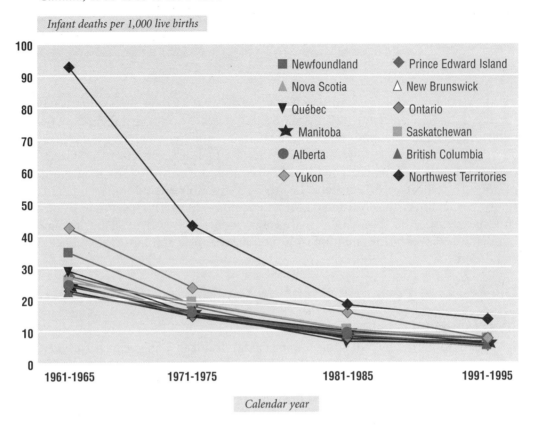

Source: Statistics Canada. Canadian Vital Statistics System, 1961-1995.

such as maternal poverty and environmental pollution were implicated in this apparent downturn in perinatal health. Others suggested a more innocuous explanation, arguing that the increase in infant mortality in 1993 was artificial and related to increases in the birth registration of live births < 500 g.[5] With previously defined limits on viability (e.g., a birth weight of 500 g) being steadily breached due to advances in obstetrics and neonatal care, attitudes towards such extremely immature live births have changed in recent years. If extremely immature live births are increasingly registered as live births, crude infant mortality comparisons over time would be compromised[5,6] as a result of the extremely high mortality among such births.[7]

This was not a new argument; the World Health Organization (WHO) recommended that international comparisons of infant mortality be restricted to live births ≥ 1,000 g for similar reasons.[8] Unfortunately, while trends in crude infant mortality rates in Canada could be assessed easily, trends in infant mortality among live births ≥ 500 g or ≥ 1,000 g could only be examined indirectly (using analyses requiring assumptions or based on statistical modeling).[5] A direct assessment of the issue was not possible, because information on birth weight-specific (or gestational age-specific) rates of infant mortality was not available in Canada.

This uncertainty is behind us. Crude infant mortality rates in Canada dropped substantially to 5.6 per 1,000 live births in 1996 and 5.5 per 1,000 live births in 1997 (see chapter 4). Furthermore, work carried out by the CPSS (along with Statistics Canada) has led to the creation of a mechanism by which information on live births and infant deaths has been linked from 1985 onwards. This linkage means that information on birth weight- and gestational age-specific infant mortality[9,10] is available for Canada and for each province/territory (see Appendix E), and that such information will become available on an ongoing basis in the future. Analyses carried out after this linkage[9] have demonstrated that crude infant mortality rates in Canada (excluding Newfoundland and Ontario) decreased by 22.1% from 8.1 per 1,000 live births in 1985-1987 to 6.3 per 1,000 live births in 1992-1994. Over the same period, infant mortality rates among live births ≥ 500 g decreased by 25.4 % (from 7.6 to 5.7 per 1,000 live births) and by 26.3% among live births ≥ 1,000 g (from 5.9 to 4.4 per 1,000 live births). The divergence between trends in crude infant mortality rates and among live births ≥ 500 g confirms that assessment of trends in infant mortality needs to account for changes in the registration of live births at the borderline of viability. Details regarding rates of fetal, neonatal, postneonatal and infant mortality in Canada and in each province/territory are provided in chapter 4 and in Appendix E.

Congenital Anomalies

One of the noteworthy changes in perinatal health in Canada in recent years has been the decline in infant deaths due to congenital malformations. Infant mortality due to major congenital anomalies decreased significantly from 3.1 per 1,000 live births in 1985 to 1.9 per 1,000 live births in 1995. The pattern of this decrease[11,12] is suggestive of increases in prenatal diagnosis and termination of affected pregnancies, coupled with improvements in the care of infants with congenital anomalies. Figure 2 shows categories of congenital anomalies which recorded substantially fewer infant deaths in recent years. Regional differences in rates of infant death due to congenital anomalies are pronounced, however.[11] Chapter 4 presents data on neural tube defects in Canada, an area of particular interest from the perinatal surveillance standpoint, given recent initiatives related to food fortification with folic acid.[13]

Infant mortality due to major congenital anomalies decreased significantly from 3.1 per 1,000 live births in 1985 to 1.9 per 1,000 live births in 1995.

Multiple Births

Multiple births have become an issue of increasing concern in Canada in recent years for two reasons: a substantial increase in the frequency of multiple births and in the rates of preterm birth among multiple birth pregnancies. Both changes are part of a long-standing trend, although the increase in frequency has accelerated in recent years (Figure 3). The frequency of multiple births increased in Canada from 18.2 per 1,000 total births in 1974 to 19.3 in 1980,[14] 20.8 in 1990 and 25.0 per 1,000 total births in 1997 (see chapter 4).

FIGURE 2
Trends in infant mortality rates due to selected congenital anomalies,
Canada (excluding British Columbia, Ontario and Newfoundland), 1981-1983 and 1993-1995

Infant deaths per 1,000 live births   ■ 1981-1983   ■ 1993-1995

1.2	
1.0	
0.8	
0.6	
0.4	
0.2	
0.0	

Anencephaly   **Other CNS**   **Respiratory**   **Musculoskeletal**   **Chromosomal**

Spina bifida   **Cardiovascular**   **Digestive**   **Urinary**   **Multiple**

Type of congenital anomaly

Source: Wen et al., 2000.[12]
CNS — central nervous system.

FIGURE 3
Rates of twin and triplet births (live and stillbirths),*
Canada, 1974-1997

■ Twins   ● Triplets

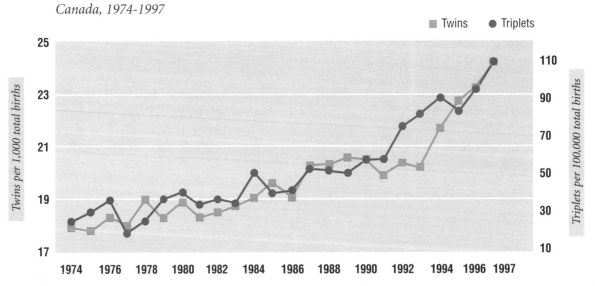

Twins per 1,000 total births   *Triplets per 100,000 total births*

Calendar year

Source: Statistics Canada. Canadian Vital Statistics System, 1974-1997.

* Rates of twin births are expressed per 1,000 total births (primary y-axis), while triplet births are per 100,000 total births (secondary y-axis).

The increase in the frequency of multiple births in Canada is paralleled by similar increases in other industrialized countries and is associated with increases in the proportion of older mothers and in infertility treatments, including pharmacologic treatments and in vitro fertilization. Insofar as these trends represent an increase in choice for women with regard to fertility and timing of pregnancy, they constitute a triumph of science and medicine. However, multiple births are associated with higher rates of fetal and infant mortality.[15-18] Serious morbidity is also higher among twins and triplets; cerebral palsy rates among triplets and twins are estimated to be 47 times and eight times higher, respectively, than among singletons.[19] As a result, triplet pregnancies are being increasingly viewed as a procedure-related complication, and a consensus is building around limits to the number of embryos transferred per in vitro fertilization cycle.[20,21]

The second concern related to multiple births is the increasing rate of preterm birth among multiple births (Figure 4). Preterm birth among multiple live births increased from 33% in 1974 to approximately 40% in 1981-1983 and 50% in 1992-1994.[22] In 1997, the rate of preterm birth among multiple live births in Canada (excluding Ontario) was 53.5% (see chapter 4). These increases in preterm birth are dramatic compared with the modest increase in preterm birth among singleton live births.[22] Preliminary studies carried out by the CPSS suggest that the increases are due to more preterm labour induction and preterm cesarean section at 34-36 weeks' gestation. These, along with various other obstetric and neonatal interventions, have resulted in reductions in fetal and infant mortality among multiple births. Nevertheless, live births at 34-36 weeks' gestation continue to contribute substantially to overall infant mortality among both singleton and multiple births.[23]

The increase in the frequency of multiple births in Canada is paralleled by similar increases in other industrialized countries and is associated with increases in the proportion of older mothers and in infertility treatments, including pharmacologic treatments and in vitro fertilization.

FIGURE 4 **Rate of preterm birth among multiple live births,**
Canada,* 1974-1997

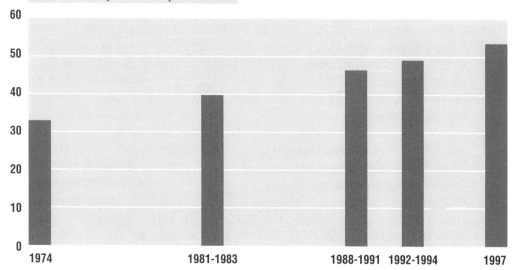

Preterm births per 100 multiple live births

Calendar year

Source: Statistics Canada. Canadian Vital Statistics System, 1974-1997.

* Data from British Columbia, Ontario and Newfoundland are not included for estimates from 1981-1994, and data from Ontario are not included for 1997 estimate.

Preterm and Postterm Birth

Rates of preterm birth have increased in Canada in recent years, whereas rates of postterm birth have declined. The increase in preterm birth, from 6.4% of all live births in 1981 to 7.1% in 1997 (see chapter 4), appears to be related to changes in multiple births, increases in obstetric intervention and the increasing use of ultrasound-based measures of gestational age.[22,24] Although preterm birth is an important determinant of perinatal mortality, the recent increases in preterm birth have been associated with declines in stillbirth rates, suggesting that obstetric intervention is largely responsible for both the increase in preterm birth and the decrease in stillbirth.[22,24] Another related trend is the improvement in fetal growth rates; temporal decreases in small-for-gestational-age live births are also described in chapter 4. These explanations do not alter the higher burden of illness implied by the increase in preterm birth, however. More importantly, it underscores our failure to reduce preterm birth, which remains the most important perinatal challenge facing industrialized countries.[25,26]

Postterm births have decreased markedly in recent years from 4.3% of total births in 1988 to 1.8% of total births in 1997 (see chapter 4); this reduction also appears to be due to obstetric intervention and changes in the modality of gestational age ascertainment. Elective labour induction is now the recommended management option for pregnancies over 41 weeks' gestation.[27] Recent Canadian studies have shown that stillbirth rates beyond term have declined as a result of increases in such labour induction, without a corresponding increase in cesarean section rates.[28] There appears to be a substantial variation in rates of postterm birth between provinces/territories, however (see chapter 4).

Maternal Health

Maternal health outcomes are described in chapter 3. The maternal mortality ratio in Canada reached 4.4 per 100,000 live births in 1993-1997 (from 8.2 per 100,000 live births in 1973-1977) and is currently one of the lowest in the world. The most common causes of maternal death in Canada are hypertensive disorders of pregnancy (9.1 per million live births in 1993-1997), pulmonary embolism (8.6 per million live births in 1993-1997), antepartum and postpartum hemorrhage (6.9 per million live births in 1993-1997) and ectopic pregnancy (4.8 per million live births in 1993-1997). The relative rarity of maternal death suggests the need for an alternative indicator of maternal health. Chapter 3 also examines issues surrounding severe maternal morbidity, as well as the rate of maternal readmission following hospital discharge after childbirth. Rates of maternal readmission following vaginal delivery (within three months after hospital discharge for reasons such as postpartum hemorrhage, cholelithiasis, puerperal infection, etc.) remained stable between 1990 and 1997 at approximately 2.5 per 100 deliveries. Maternal readmission rates following cesarean delivery increased slightly from 3.2 in 1990 to 3.9 per 100 deliveries in 1997, however. Maternal readmission rates after childbirth among those delivering by cesarean section have been shown to be associated with a short hospital stay (< 2 days versus 5 days),[29] suggesting that the practice of sending women home soon after delivery by cesarean section needs closer examination.

Preterm birth remains the most important perinatal challenge facing industrialized countries.

In 1989, episiotomies were performed on 55% of women who delivered vaginally. By 1997, this rate had decreased to 25%. Sharply decreasing trends in episiotomy rates (see chapter 2) are in keeping with recent evidence in the medical literature that routine use of episiotomy may not be justified and consequent changes in obstetric practice. Rates of severe perineal lacerations remained stable over this period.

Behaviours and Practices in Pregnancy

A number of behaviours and practices during pregnancy and after childbirth are outlined in chapter 1. The rate of breastfeeding initiation (and the duration of breastfeeding) varied widely across Canada, with the highest rates of breastfeeding initiation present in western parts of the country (58% in Québec versus 89% in British Columbia). On average, approximately 77% of children born in Canada in the mid-1990s were breastfed for some duration. The east-to-west gradient was also apparent in rates of maternal cigarette smoking, with 25% of mothers in the Atlantic Provinces and Québec smoking during pregnancy, as compared with 19% in British Columbia. Information on alcohol consumption during pregnancy is also provided in chapter 1. Also documented are increasing rates of birth among older mothers and relatively low and stable rates of live births to teenage mothers.

Health Service Issues

Labour induction, operative vaginal delivery and cesarean section rates are presented in chapter 2. The recent increase in cesarean section rates (from 17.8% in 1994 to 19.1% in 1997) was due to increases in primary cesarean section rates, and an argument is made in chapter 2 that examining trends in crude rates of cesarean section is helpful only if changes in parity and maternal age are considered simultaneously. The rate of operative vaginal delivery varied widely between the provinces and territories in 1997. Forceps deliveries ranged from a low of less than 3 per 100 vaginal deliveries in hospitals in the territories and in Manitoba to a high of about 8 per 100 vaginal deliveries among hospitals in New Brunswick, Newfoundland, Nova Scotia and Ontario. Vacuum deliveries were least common in the Northwest Territories, Nova Scotia and Prince Edward Island (4-5 per 100 vaginal deliveries in hospital), and most frequent in Saskatchewan and the Yukon (14-15 per 100 vaginal deliveries in hospital).

Substantial changes in health care services have occurred in Canada in recent years, including reductions in the neonatal and maternal length of hospital stay following childbirth. The proportion of newborns and mothers discharged from hospital after a short stay following birth, trends over time and interprovincial/territorial variations have been described previously,[30,31] and updates are presented in chapter 2. In 1997, approximately 29% of normal birth weight newborns were discharged from hospital within two days following birth (up from 3.1% in 1989). Similarly, short hospital stays for mothers have also increased following both vaginal delivery (3.2% stayed < 2 days in 1989 versus 25.6% in 1997) and delivery by cesarean section (2.1% stayed < 4 days in 1989 versus 25.6% in 1997). The consequences of these trends in terms of changes in readmission rates for mothers and babies have also been documented previously,[32,33] and recent information is presented in chapters 3 and 4.

The rate of breastfeeding initiation (and the duration of breastfeeding) varies widely across Canada, with the highest rates of breastfeeding initiation present in Western parts of the country.

On average, approximately 77% of children born in Canada in the mid-1990s were breastfed for some duration.

A Framework for Action

Benchmarking as a Strategy for Improving Perinatal Health

A framework of surveillance which uses benchmarking to identify rates of excess mortality and direct public health efforts is described in chapter 4. The premise is that if one segment of the population has achieved a high standard of health in a particular domain, improvements in that dimension of health are possible for other populations as well. Benchmark rates of birth weight-specific fetal and infant mortality were estimated among mothers in Québec who had high levels of education (since education is known to positively influence perinatal outcomes).[34] The benchmark population chosen was identified within Québec, as it was the only province with information on the educational status of all mothers. Birth weight-specific rates of fetal and infant mortality were then calculated for each province and territory and compared with the benchmark to identify excess rates of mortality. The categorization of deaths by birth weight and age at death permits broad generalizations to be made about the particular components of maternal and child health that may be responsible for excess mortality (e.g., maternal care versus newborn care).

The appeal of this approach to surveillance is that it provides the health system with a clear direction for decentralized program evaluation, program planning and public health action. For instance, high rates of fetal mortality among births ≥ 1,500 g in a province/territory (relative to the benchmark) suggest that maternal care issues need to be examined in that region. The excess fetal deaths could be indicative of problems with timely access to high quality obstetric care (especially in rural areas). However, excess mortality may also be due to other factors, including differences in rates of specific behaviours in pregnancy. A careful investigation can build on the information in this report, identify the issues responsible for excess mortality in a region and help direct public health policy so that it has maximum impact on the subpopulation most in need of attention.

Areas of Perinatal Health Concern

Although the current state of perinatal health in Canada is better than it has been in previous years, some disparities between subpopulations persist. Despite access to universal health care, socio-economic status remains a determinant of perinatal health.

Although the current state of perinatal health in Canada is better than it has been in previous years, some disparities between subpopulations persist. Despite universal health insurance, socioeconomic status remains a determinant of perinatal health. Infant mortality rates among the lowest income groups in urban Canada were two-fold higher than infant mortality rates among the highest income groups in 1971.[35] This difference appears to have been slightly attenuated but not eliminated two decades later; low income groups experienced a 1.6 times greater risk of infant death compared with high income groups in 1991.[36]

Perinatal health among the First Nations, Métis and Inuit populations needs particular attention. The rates of stillbirth and perinatal mortality among registered Indians have been estimated to be about double the Canadian average, while rates among the Inuit in the Northwest Territories are about two and a half times the rates for Canada as a whole.[37] Similarly, infant mortality rates among registered Indians and the Inuit were estimated to be approximately 14 and 20 per 1,000 live births, respectively (while infant mortality rates were 7 per 1,000 live births for Canada as a whole).[37] Studies have shown[38] that deaths due to sudden infant death syndrome among First Nations infants (relative to other infants) were five times higher in British Columbia and 10 times as high in Alberta.

Addressing these perinatal disparities represents a challenge for Canada ("a test of its national character")[39] for various reasons, including the need to delineate the proper approach to health promotion in the context of Aboriginal culture and empowerment.[39]

Crude infant mortality rates in Saskatchewan have shown an unexpected trend over the last decade, increasing from 7.6 (95% confidence interval 6.4 to 9.1) per 1,000 live births in 1990[40] to 8.9 (95% confidence interval 7.3 to 10.6) per 1,000 live births in 1997 (see chapter 4). Rates in Canada as a whole declined from 6.8 to 5.5 per 1,000 live births over the same period. However, this phenomenon was identified at an early stage and provincial initiatives to address this issue are under way in Saskatchewan.

Regional differences in the use of various medical procedures (i.e., inter-provincial/territorial differences in the use of forceps/vacuum, differences in rates of postterm birth, etc.) require consideration from the obstetric community, as well as further study. Temporal trends of concern include small but significant increases in neonatal hospital readmission and maternal hospital readmission following childbirth by cesarean section. These trends imply that the policy towards short hospital stays for mothers and newborns needs to be refined through improved routine assessment of patients prior to hospital discharge.

Maternal smoking, alcohol consumption during pregnancy and breastfeeding initiation/duration are priority areas of social and public health concern. The absolute rates of these indicators and regional differences in rates underscore the need for additional supportive public health programs designed to inform women about the effects of particular behaviours in pregnancy. Beyond providing information and creating a social climate which encourages healthy behaviours, public health programs also face the challenge of supporting and helping women who are addicted to harmful behaviours.

Areas for Improvement in Perinatal Health Surveillance

Much of the information in this report provides a generally accurate picture of the current perinatal health situation in Canada. For example, the relatively high rate of postterm birth in Nova Scotia in 1997 (4.7% of total births; see chapter 4) obtained from the Discharge Abstract Database (DAD) of the Canadian Institute for Health Information (CIHI) concurs with a similar rate obtained from the Nova Scotia Atlee Perinatal Database (4.2% of all deliveries).[41]

Some of the regional variation identified in this report may be due to chance or differences in data quality, however. Sifting through the information, correlating it with regional information from other sources and identifying potential errors will, over time, help to improve the quality of perinatal surveillance in Canada. We have completed a preliminary examination of the discrepancy between rates of respiratory distress syndrome (RDS) in Nova Scotia obtained from CIHI data (10.7 per 1,000 live births in 1997, see chapter 4) and from the Nova Scotia Atlee Perinatal Database (18.2 per 1,000 live births in 1997).[41] A validation study of CIHI data and a closer examination of potential discrepencies in information are under way.

This report clearly identifies several areas where surveillance information is insufficient for the purpose of quantifying and fully understanding the state of perinatal health in this country. Inadequacies include areas where little or no information is available for Canada as a whole (e.g., on the use of assisted reproduction), areas where routine information is not collected (e.g., parity in

Efforts are being made to increase the content of national vital statistics and hospital discharge databases so as to better serve perinatal health surveillance. The ultimate goal of these efforts is the creation of a national database that captures information critical for perinatal surveillance in a timely manner.

relation to cesarean section rates, on behaviours and experiences in pregnancy and in the postpartum period, including maternal drug use and postpartum depression) and areas where the quality of routine information is inadequate (e.g., the province of Ontario in previous years). The lack of routine surveillance information on Aboriginal Canadians also indicates a serious gap in the current system of perinatal health surveillance in Canada.

The CPSS is attempting to address some of these shortcomings through various initiatives. Efforts are being made, in conjunction with Statistics Canada and the CIHI, to increase the content of national vital statistics and hospital discharge databases so as to better serve perinatal health surveillance. The ultimate goal of these efforts is the creation of a national database that captures information critical for perinatal surveillance in a timely manner. Another initiative involves conducting regular surveys in order to document important behaviours and practices during pregnancy. Efforts are also ongoing, in conjunction with Statistics Canada and the First Nations and Inuit Health Branch of Health Canada, to develop a national system which routinely reports on First Nations and Inuit fetal and infant mortality. The creation of a common perinatal clinical record for collecting standardized information across Canada is also a long-term goal. However, these initiatives should be viewed as complementary to regional efforts to improve data quality and increase the amount of detailed information collected. Such independent efforts will allow regional health systems to identify local issues more quickly, explore areas of regional concern and better respond to disparities identified by national level surveillance.

A system of high quality perinatal health surveillance is critical to understanding and improving perinatal health.

Conclusion

This surveillance report highlights various components of perinatal health in Canada. By identifying trends over recent years and reporting on regional differences, it provides useful information that can be utilized by practitioners and policy makers to further improve perinatal health. The report also highlights gaps in perinatal health information. Although efforts are under way to address these deficiencies, this report will spur on greater progress in data collection, analysis and interpretation by highlighting both the strengths and weaknesses of perinatal health surveillance in Canada.

A system of high quality perinatal health surveillance is critical to understanding and improving perinatal health. Although the information presented in this report confirms the enviable status of perinatal health in Canada from a global perspective, several specific areas of perinatal health are identified as needing further support. Both public health programs and those working in the field of perinatal health will benefit from the information contained in this report.

K.S. Joseph, MD, PhD
Assistant Professor
Perinatal Epidemiology Research Unit
Departments of Obstetrics and Gynecology and Pediatrics
Dalhousie University, Halifax, Nova Scotia
Member, Steering Committee of the Canadian Perinatal Surveillance System

References

1. Dzakpasu S, Joseph KS, Kramer MS, Allen AC. The Matthew Effect: infant mortality in Canada and internationally. *Pediatrics* 2000; 106: e5.

2. Howell EM, Blondel B. International infant mortality rates: bias from reporting differences. *Am J Public Health* 1994; 84: 850-2.

3. Sepkowitz S. International rankings of infant mortality and the United States vital statistics natality data collecting system — failure and success. *Int J Epidemiol* 1995; 24: 583-8.

4. Mitchell A. Rising deaths among infants stun scientists. *Globe and Mail* [Toronto]. June 2, 1995: A4.

5. Joseph KS, Kramer MS. Recent trends in Canadian infant mortality rates: Effect of changes in registration of live newborns weighing less than 500 grams. *Can Med Assoc J* 1996; 155: 1047-52.

6. Svenson LW, Schopflocher DP, Sauve RS, Robertson CM. Alberta's infant mortality rate: the effect of the registration of live newborns weighing less than 500 g. *Can J Public Health* 1998; 89: 188-9.

7. Sauve RS, Robertson C, Etches P, Byrne PJ, Dayer-Zamora V. Before viability: a geographically based outcome study of infants weighing 500 grams or less at birth. *Pediatrics* 1998; 101: 438-45.

8. World Health Organization. *International Statistical Classification of Diseases and Related Health Problems*, 10th Revision. Vol. 2. Geneva: WHO, 1993: 129-33.

9. Joseph KS, Kramer MS, Allen AC, Cyr M, Fair M, Ohlsson A et al. for the Fetal-Infant Mortality Study Group of the Canadian Perinatal Surveillance System. Gestational age- and birth weight-specific declines in infant mortality in Canada, 1985-94. *Paediatr Perinat Epidemiol* (in press).

10. Wen SW, Kramer MS, Liu S, Dzakpasu S, Sauve R for the Fetal and Infant Health Study Group. Infant mortality by gestational age and birth weight in Canadian provinces and territories, 1990-1994 births. *Chronic Dis Can* 2000; 21: 14-22.

11. Wen SW, Liu S, Joseph KS, Trouton K, Allen A. Regional patterns of infant mortality caused by lethal congenital anomalies. *Can J Public Health* 1999; 90: 316-9.

12. Wen SW, Liu S, Joseph KS, Rouleau J, Allen A. Patterns of infant mortality caused by major congenital anomalies. *Teratology* 2000; 61: 342-6.

13. Turner LA, McCourt C. Folic acid fortification: what does it mean for patients and physicians? *Can Med Assoc J* 1998; 158: 773-6.

14. Millar WJ, Wadhera S, Nimrod C. Multiple births: trends and patterns in Canada, 1974-90. *Health Rep* 1992; 4: 223-50.

15. Kallen B. Congenital malformations in twins: a population study. *Acta Genet Med Gemello Roma* 1986; 35: 167-78.

16. Rodis JF, Egan JF, Craffey A, Ciarleglio L, Greenstein RM, Scorza WE. Calculated risk of chromosomal abnormalities in twin gestations. *Obstet Gynecol* 1990; 76: 1037-41.

17. Bryan EM. The intrauterine hazards of twins. *Arch Dis Child* 1986; 61: 1044-5.

18. Grobman WA, Peaceman AM. What are the rates and mechanisms of first and second trimester pregnancy loss in twins? *Clin Obstet Gynecol* 1998; 41: 37-45.

19. Petterson B, Nelson KB, Watson L, Stanley F. Twins, triplets, and cerebral palsy in births in Western Australia in the 1980's. *Br Med J* 1993; 307: 1239-43.

20. Fisk NM, Trew G. Two's company, three's a crowd for embryo transfer *Lancet* 1999; 354. 1572-3.

21. Society of Obstetricians and Gynaecologists of Canada. *The SOGC consensus statement on the management of twin pregnancies. Part two: Report of focus group on impact of twin pregnancies.* Barrett J. (Ed.). (Available: www.sogc.org/multiple/sogcconsensus.htm)

22. Joseph KS, Kramer MS, Marcoux S, Ohlsson A, Wen SW, Allen A et al. Determinants of preterm birth rates in Canada from 1981 through 1983 and from 1992 through 1994. *N Engl J Med* 1998; 339: 1434-9.

23. Kramer MS, Demissie K, Yang H, Platt RW, Sauve R, Liston R for the Fetal and Infant Health Study Group of the Canadian Perinatal Surveillance System. The contribution of mild and moderate preterm birth to infant mortality. *J Am Med Assoc* 2000; 284: 843-9.

24. Kramer MS, Platt R, Yang H, Joseph KS, Wen SW, Morin L et al. Secular trends in preterm birth: A hospital-based cohort study. *J Am Med Assoc* 1998; 280: 1849-54.

25. Morrison JC. Preterm birth: a puzzle worth solving. *Obstet Gynecol* 1990; 76: 5S-12S.

26. Creasy RK, Merkatz IR. Prevention of preterm birth: clinical opinion. *Obstet Gynecol* 1990; 76: 2S-4S.

27. Crowley P. Interventions for preventing or improving the outcome of delivery at or beyond term (Cochrane Review). In: *The Cochrane Library, Issue 1*. Oxford: Update Software, 2000.

28. Sue-A-Quan AK, Hannah ME, Cohen MM, Foster GA, Liston RM. Effect of labour induction on rates of stillbirth and cesarean section in post-term pregnancies. *Can Med Assoc J* 1999; 160: 1145-9.

29. Liu S, Heaman M, Kramer MS, Demissie K, Turner L for the Maternal Mortality and Morbidity Study Group of the Canadian Perinatal Surveillance System. Association between length of hospital stay, obstetric conditions at childbirth, and maternal rehospitalization [submitted for publication].

30. Wen SW, Liu S, Marcoux S, Fowler D. Trends and variations in length of hospital stay for childbirth in Canada. *Can Med Assoc J* 1998: 158: 875-80.

31. Wen SW, Liu S, Fowler D. Trends and variations in neonatal length of in-hospital stay in Canada. *Can J Public Health* 1998; 89: 115-9.

32. Liu S, Wen SW, McMillan D, Trouton K, Fowler D, McCourt C. Increased neonatal readmission rate associated with decreased length of hospital stay at birth in Canada. *Can J Public Health* 2000; 91: 46-50.

33. Liu S, Heaman M, Demissie K, Wen SW, Marcoux S, Kramer MS. Association between maternal readmission and obstetric conditions at childbirth: a case-control study. Presented at the 13th Annual Meeting of the Society for Pediatric and Perinatal Epidemiologic Research, Seattle, Washington, June 2000.

34. Chen J, Fair M, Wilkins R, Cyr M and the Fetal and Infant Mortality Study Group of the Canadian Perinatal Surveillance System. Maternal education and fetal and infant mortality in Quebec. *Health Rep* 1998; 10: 53-64.

35. Wilkins R, Adams O, Branker A. Changes in mortality by income in urban Canada from 1971 to 1986. *Health Rep* 1989; 1: 137-74.

36. Wilkins R. Mortality by neighbourhood income in urban Canada, 1986-1991. Presentation at the Canadian Society for Epidemiology and Biostatistics, Newfoundland, Canada, August 1995.

37. *Final Report of the Royal Commission on Aboriginal Peoples*. Ottawa, 1996. (Available: www.inac.gc.ca/ch/rcap/index_e.html).

38. *SIDS Fact Sheet*. Assembly of First Nations. National Indian Brotherhood 2000. (Available: www.afn.ca/Programs/Health%20Secretariat/sids_fact_sheet.htm).

39. Postl B. Native health: it's time for action. *Can Med Assoc J* 1997; 157: 165-6.

40. Canadian Centre for Health Information. *Births 1990*. Ottawa: Statistics Canada, 1992 (Catalogue No. 82-003S14).

41. Reproductive Care Program of Nova Scotia. *Nova Scotia Atlee Perinatal Database Report: Maternal and Infant Discharges from January 1-December 31, 1997*. Halifax: 2000.

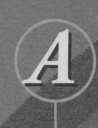

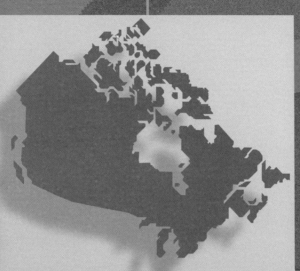

Determinants of Maternal, Fetal and Infant Health

Behaviours and Practices

Prevalence of Prenatal Smoking

The prevalence of prenatal smoking is defined as the number of pregnant women who smoked cigarettes during pregnancy expressed as a proportion of all pregnant women (in a given place and time).

Prenatal cigarette smoking can have adverse health effects on the fetus and child. It increases the risk of intrauterine growth restriction (IUGR), preterm birth, spontaneous abortion and stillbirth.[1-4] It also increases the risk of sudden infant death syndrome and has been associated with impaired physical and intellectual development of the child. Prenatal smoking is related to an overall increased risk of infant mortality and morbidity, due in part to increases in IUGR and preterm birth.

The relationship between prenatal smoking and adverse pregnancy outcomes is linked to the amount and duration of smoking. Women who stop smoking before becoming pregnant or during the first trimester of pregnancy are at significantly reduced risk of having a low birth weight baby compared with women who smoke throughout pregnancy.[4] Although pregnant women are more likely to quit smoking and smoke fewer cigarettes than women who are not pregnant, prenatal smoking remains an important public health problem. It is important to continue to promote non-smoking among women in general, and to help smoking women who become pregnant to stop smoking as early as possible.

Since there are no data on prenatal smoking for all pregnancies in Canada, rates were estimated using the 1996-1997 National Longitudinal Survey of Children and Youth (NLSCY).

Although pregnant women are more likely to quit smoking and smoke fewer cigarettes than women who are not pregnant, prenatal smoking remains an important public health problem.

Results

- In Canada in 1996-1997, 21.3% of children under the age of three had mothers who reported smoking during their pregnancy. Seven percent reported smoking more than 10 cigarettes per day. Among smokers, 90.9% reported smoking in the third trimester of pregnancy, when the negative effect on fetal growth is greatest.

- Younger mothers were more likely to report smoking. In 1996-1997, 40.5% (this estimate was based on a small sample) of children whose mothers were under 20 years of age were exposed to tobacco prenatally, compared with 17.2% of children whose mothers were 35 years or older (Figure 1.1). This inverse relationship between smoking and age is also present in the general (non-pregnant) Canadian female population.

- Reported rates of prenatal smoking varied by region. Rates ranged from lows of 18.6% and 18.8% in British Columbia and Ontario, respectively, to highs of 25.8% in Québec and 25.2% in the Atlantic Provinces (Figure 1.2).

FIGURE 1.1 **Prevalence of prenatal smoking, by maternal age,**
Canada (excluding the territories), 1996-1997*

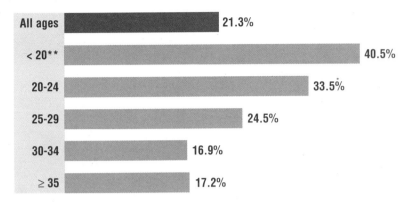

All ages — 21.3%
< 20** — 40.5%
20-24 — 33.5%
25-29 — 24.5%
30-34 — 16.9%
≥ 35 — 17.2%

Percent of children 0-3 years old whose mothers reported smoking prenatally

Source: Statistics Canada. National Longitudinal Survey of Children and Youth (Public Use Microdata Files), 1996-1997.
* Data for the territories are not available in the Public Use Microdata Files.
** Estimate for this age group is based on a small sample size.

FIGURE 1.2 **Prevalence of prenatal smoking, by region/province,**
Canada (excluding the territories), 1996-1997*

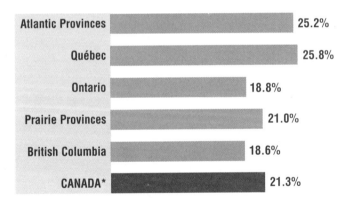

Atlantic Provinces — 25.2%
Québec — 25.8%
Ontario — 18.8%
Prairie Provinces — 21.0%
British Columbia — 18.6%
CANADA* — 21.3%

Percent of children 0-3 years old whose mothers reported smoking prenatally

Source: Statistics Canada. National Longitudinal Survey of Children and Youth (Public Use Microdata Files), 1996-1997.
* Data for the territories are not available in the Public Use Microdata Files.

Data Limitations

The knowledge that smoking during pregnancy can adversely affect the outcome of the pregnancy may have led mothers to under-report their smoking behaviour during pregnancy.[5] Therefore, rates of prenatal smoking in Canada are probably higher than those reported in the NLSCY.

References

1. Edwards N, Sims-Jones N, Hotz S. *Pre and Postnatal Smoking: A Review of the Literature.* Ottawa: Health Canada, 1996.

2. Werler MM. Teratogen update: smoking and reproductive outcomes. *Teratology* 1997; 55: 382-8.

3. Tuormaa TE. The adverse effects of tobacco smoking on reproduction and health: a review from the literature. *Nutr Health* 1995; 10: 105-20.

4. U.S. Department of Health and Human Services. *The Health Benefits of Smoking Cessation.* U.S. Department of Health and Human Services, Public Health Service, Centers for Disease Control, Center for Chronic Disease Prevention and Health Promotion, Office of Smoking and Health, 1990 (DHHS Publication No. (CDC) 90-8416).

5. Patrick DL, Cheadle A, Thompson DC, Diehr P, Koepsell T, Kinne S. The validity of self-reported smoking: a review and meta analysis. *Am J Public Health* 1994; 84: 1086-93.

Prevalence of Prenatal Alcohol Consumption

In Canada in 1996-1997, 16.6% of children under the age of three had mothers who reported drinking alcohol during pregnancy.

The prevalence of prenatal alcohol consumption is defined as the number of pregnant women who consumed alcoholic beverages during pregnancy expressed as a proportion of all pregnant women (in a given place and time).

Prenatal alcohol consumption can result in alcohol-related birth defects (ARBD). ARBDs exhibit a continuum of severity, with spontaneous abortion, intrauterine growth restriction (IUGR) and fetal alcohol syndrome (FAS) being among the more severe effects.[1-3] Other effects include cognitive and behavioural abnormalities, which can persist into adulthood and significantly impair an individual's quality of life. The effects of prenatal alcohol consumption are thought to depend on a number of factors, including the quantity of alcohol consumed, the stage(s) during pregnancy when the alcohol is consumed, the mother's ability to metabolize alcohol and the genetic makeup of the fetus.[1,2] However, since a safe level of alcohol consumption during pregnancy has not been determined, Health Canada recommends that women abstain from alcohol consumption if they are pregnant or planning to become pregnant.[3]

Since there are no data on prenatal alcohol consumption for all pregnancies in Canada, rates were estimated using the 1996-1997 National Longitudinal Survey of Children and Youth (NLSCY).

Results

- In Canada in 1996-1997, 16.6% of children under the age of three had mothers who reported drinking alcohol during pregnancy. This percentage includes all mothers who reported drinking, regardless of amount. ARBDs are likely related to chronic, heavy alcohol exposure, rather than low, steady rates of drinking.[4,5] Unfortunately, the proportion of children with chronic, heavy prenatal alcohol exposure could not be determined reliably using NLSCY data.

- Older mothers were more likely to report prenatal alcohol consumption. In 1996-1997, 11.7% of children whose mothers were under 25 years of age were exposed to some alcohol prenatally compared with 22.6% of children whose mothers were 35 years and older (Figure 1.3). However, previous studies have suggested that binge drinking (consumption of five or more drinks per occasion) may be more prevalent among younger women.[6]

- Reported rates of prenatal alcohol consumption varied by region. Rates ranged from a low of 7.7% in the Atlantic Provinces (this estimate was based on a small sample) to a high of 24.9% in Québec (Figure 1.4).

FIGURE 1.3 **Prevalence of prenatal alcohol consumption, by maternal age,**
Canada (excluding the territories),* 1996-1997

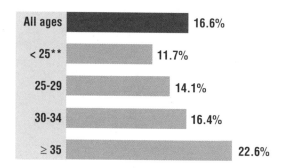

Percent of children 0-3 years old whose mothers reported drinking alcohol prenatally

Source: Statistics Canada. National Longitudinal Survey of Children and Youth (Public Use Microdata Files), 1996-1997.
* Data for the territories are not available in the Public Use Microdata Files.
** Further categorization of age was not possible due to a small sample size.

FIGURE 1.4 **Prevalence of prenatal alcohol consumption, by region/province,**
Canada (excluding the territories),* 1996-1997

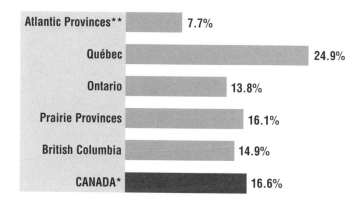

Percent of children 0-3 years old whose mothers reported drinking alcohol prenatally

Source: Statistics Canada. National Longitudinal Survey of Children and Youth (Public Use Microdata Files), 1996-1997.
* Data for the territories are not available in the Public Use Microdata Files.
** Estimate for the Atlantic Provinces is based on a small sample size.

Data Limitations

There may be systematic under-reporting of maternal alcohol consumption in surveys, because prenatal alcohol consumption is considered socially undesirable and known to incur risk to the fetus.[7] Therefore, rates of prenatal alcohol consumption are probably higher than those reported in the NLSCY.

References

1. Abel EL (Ed.). *Fetal Alcohol Syndrome, from Mechanism to Prevention.* New York: CRC Press, 1996.

2. Huebert K, Rafts C. *Fetal Alcohol Syndrome and Other Alcohol Related Birth Defects*, 2nd Edition. Edmonton: Alberta Alcohol and Drug Abuse Commission, 1996.

3. Health Canada. *Joint Statement: Prevention of Fetal Alcohol Syndrome (FAS), Fetal Alcohol Effects (FAE) in Canada.* Ottawa: Health Canada, October 1996 (Catalogue No. H39-348/1996E).

4. Abel EL. "Moderate" drinking during pregnancy: cause for concern? *Clin Chim Acta* 1996; 246: 149-54.

5. Gladstone J, Nulman I, Koren G. Reproductive risks of binge drinking during pregnancy. *Reprod Toxicol* 1996; 10: 3-13.

6. Gladstone J, Levy M, Nulman I, Koren G. Characteristics of pregnant women who engage in binge alcohol consumption. *Can Med Assoc J* 1997; 156: 789-94.

7. Stoler JM, Huntington KS, Peterson CM, Peterson KP, Daniel P, Aboagye KK et al. The prenatal detection of significant alcohol exposure with maternal blood markers. *J Pediatr* 1998; 133: 346-52.

Prevalence of Breastfeeding

The prevalence of breastfeeding is defined as the number of women who delivered and ever breastfed a live born child expressed as a proportion of all women who delivered a live born child (in a given place and time).

There is compelling evidence that breastfeeding is beneficial to infants and mothers. Human milk protects the infant from gastrointestinal and respiratory infections and otitis media, and has also been associated with enhanced cognitive development.[1-3] Beneficial effects for mothers associated with breastfeeding include reduced postpartum bleeding and delayed resumption of ovulation which helps to increase the spacing between pregnancies. There is also evidence that lactating women have improved postpartum bone remineralization and a reduced risk of ovarian and breast cancers.[1,2]

Breastfeeding prevalence rates in Canada were estimated using data from the 1996-1997 National Longitudinal Survey of Children and Youth (NLSCY).

Results

- In Canada in 1996-1997, 76.7% of children under the age of three had been breastfed for some period of time. Among children between the ages of three months and three years, 53.6% had been breastfed for at least three months. The Canadian Paediatric Society (CPS), Dieticians of Canada (DC) and Health Canada recommend exclusive breastfeeding for at least the first four months of life, and continuing breastfeeding and complementary foods for up to two years of age and beyond.[2]

- Breastfeeding initiation rates varied slightly by maternal age. Rates among mothers 30 years and older were slightly higher compared with rates among younger mothers (Figure 1.5). Breastfeeding duration also increased with increasing maternal age. Among children between the ages of three months and three years, only 31.6% born to mothers less than 20 years of age were breastfed for at least three months, compared with 59.2% of children whose mothers were 35 years or older.

- Breastfeeding initiation varied by region, with rates ranging from a low of 57.7% in Québec to highs of 89.0% in British Columbia and 88.0% in the Prairie Provinces (Figure 1.6). Mothers in regions with higher breastfeeding initiation rates also tended to breastfeed for a longer duration. In Québec, only 34.8% of children between three months and three years old were breastfed for at least three months compared with 65.2% in British Columbia.

Data Limitations

The NLSCY did not ask mothers if breastfeeding was exclusive.

There is compelling evidence that breastfeeding is beneficial to infants and mothers. Human milk protects the infant from gastrointestinal and respiratory infections and otitis media, and has also been associated with enhanced cognitive development.

FIGURE 1.5 **Prevalence of breastfeeding, by maternal age,**
Canada (excluding the territories),* 1996-1997

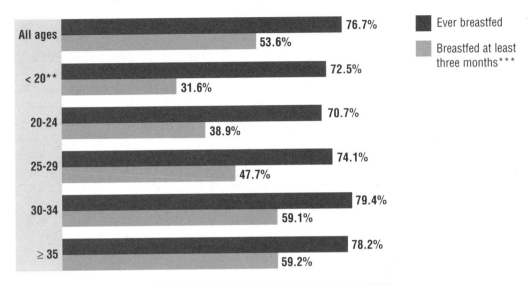

Percent of children 0-3 years old whose mothers reported breastfeeding

Source: Statistics Canada. National Longitudinal Survey of Children and Youth (Public Use Microdata Files), 1996-1997.
* Data for the territories are not available in the Public Use Microdata Files.
** Estimate of the proportion of children breastfed for at least three months is based on a small sample size.
*** Children less than three months old were excluded from "breastfed at least three months" calculations.

FIGURE 1.6 **Prevalence of breastfeeding, by region/province,**
Canada (excluding the territories),* 1996-1997

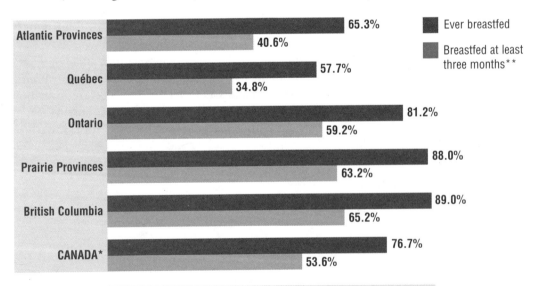

Percent of children 0-3 years old whose mothers reported breastfeeding

Source: Statistics Canada. National Longitudinal Survey of Children and Youth (Public Use Microdata Files), 1996-1997.
* Data for the territories are not available in the Public Use Microdata Files.
** Children less than three months old were excluded from "breastfed at least three months" calculations.

References

1. American Academy of Pediatrics, Work Group on Breastfeeding. Breastfeeding and the use of human milk. *Pediatrics* 1997; 100: 1035-9.

2. Canadian Paediatric Society, Dieticians of Canada and Health Canada. *Nutrition for Healthy Term Infants.* Ottawa: Minister of Public Works and Government Services Canada, 1998.

3. Breastfeeding Committee for Canada. *Breastfeeding Statement of the Breastfeeding Committee for Canada,* 1996.

Rate of Live Births to Teenage Mothers

T he age-specific live birth rate for teenage mothers is defined as the number of live births to mothers aged 10-14 or 15-19 years per 1,000 females in the same age category (in a given place and time). A related indicator is the proportion of live births to teenage mothers which refers to the number of live births to mothers aged 10-14 or 15-19 years expressed as a percentage of all live births (in a given place and time).

Various adverse maternal and infant effects of teenage pregnancy have been documented in the scientific literature, including biological and social effects. Typically, teen pregnancies are characterized by delayed entry into prenatal care and lower rates of prenatal care. Tobacco, alcohol and other substance abuse is reported to be higher among pregnant adolescents.[1] A relatively higher proportion of teenagers report physical and sexual abuse during pregnancy. Compared with mothers 20-24 years of age, mothers aged 17 years or less have an increased risk for delivering babies who are preterm or growth restricted.[2] Other adverse outcomes associated with teen pregnancies include preeclampsia, anemia, urinary tract infection and postpartum hemorrhage.[3]

Rates of live births to teenage mothers were calculated using vital statistics data.

Compared with mothers 20-24 years of age, mothers aged 17 years or less have an increased risk for delivering babies who are preterm or growth restricted.

Results

- Since 1981, the age-specific live birth rate among teenagers 10-14 years of age has declined slightly from a high of 0.29 per 1,000 teenagers of the same age to 0.22 per 1,000 in 1997 (Figure 1.7).

- For older teenagers (aged 15-19 years), the age-specific live birth rate showed peaks in the early 1980s and again in the early 1990s (Figure 1.8). The peak in the early 1990s was also observed in the U.S.[4] Since 1991, the live birth rate for teens 15-19 years of age has declined to a low of 19.9 births per 1,000 females in 1997.

- In 1997, 5.6% of all live births in Canada were to women aged 15-19 years of age, an absolute decline of 2.5% since 1981 (Figure 1.9). Live births to females less than 15 years of age account for less than 1% of all live births in Canada.

Data Limitations

Canadian data on maternal age are obtained from birth certificates and are unstated in a small fraction of records. Late registered births, stillbirths, ectopic pregnancies and aborted pregnancies are not included in the above statistics.

FIGURE 1.7 **Age-specific live birth rate, females 10-14 years,**
Canada (excluding Newfoundland),* 1981-1997

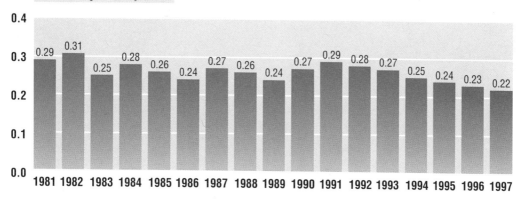

Live births per 1,000 females

Sources: Statistics Canada. Canadian Vital Statistics System, 1981-1997.
Statistics Canada. Canadian female population estimates, 1981-1997.
* Newfoundland is excluded because data are not available nationally prior to 1991.

FIGURE 1.8 **Age-specific live birth rate, females 15-19 years,**
Canada (excluding Newfoundland),* 1981-1997

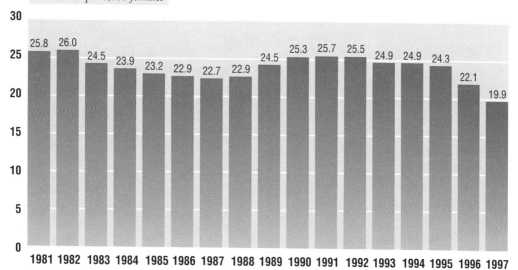

Live births per 1,000 females

Sources: Statistics Canada. Canadian Vital Statistics System, 1981-1997.
Statistics Canada. Canadian female population estimates, 1981-1997.
* Newfoundland is excluded because data are not available nationally prior to 1991.

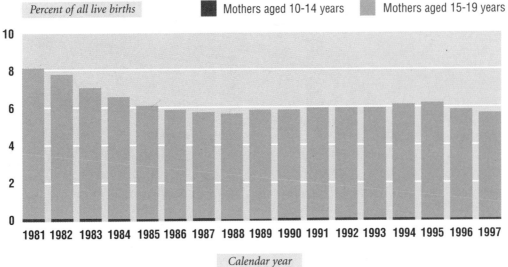

FIGURE 1.9 **Percent of live births to teenage mothers,**
Canada (excluding Newfoundland), 1981-1997*

Source: Statistics Canada. Canadian Vital Statistics System, 1981-1997.
* Newfoundland is excluded because data are not available nationally prior to 1991.

References

1. Huizinga D, Loeber R, Thornberry TP. Longitudinal study of delinquency, drug use, sexual activity and pregnancy among children and youth in three cities. *Public Health Rep* 1993; 108 (S1): 90-6.

2. Fraser AM, Brockert JE, Ward RH. Association of young maternal age with adverse reproductive outcomes. *N Engl J Med* 1995; 332: 1113-7.

3. Miller HS, Lesser KB, Reed KL. Adolescence and very low birth weight infants: A disproportionate association. *Obstet Gynecol* 1996; 87: 83-8.

4. Ventura SJ, Martin JA, Curtin SC, Mathews TJ. Births: Final Data for 1997. *National vital statistics reports*; vol 47, no. 18. Hyattsville, Maryland: National Center for Health Statistics, 1999.

Rate of Live Births to Older Mothers

The age-specific live birth rate for older mothers is defined as the number of live births to women aged 30-34, 35-39, 40-44 or 45 years and older per 1,000 women in the same age category (in a given place and time). A related indicator is the proportion of live births to older mothers which refers to the number of live births to mothers aged 30-34, 35-39, 40-44 or 45 years and older expressed as a percentage of all live births (in a given place and time).

The proportion of women who are delaying childbearing to later years has increased markedly in Canada in recent years. There is some evidence that this may be associated with adverse outcomes to both mother and infant. For example, the frequency of Down's syndrome increases with advancing maternal age from less than 1 per 1,000 births at age 20 years to 2.5-3.9 per 1,000 at age 35 years, 8.5-13.7 per 1,000 at age 40 years and 28.7-52.3 per 1,000 births at age 45 years.[1] Antepartum complications shown to be associated with delayed childbearing include increased risks for spontaneous abortion, gestational diabetes, prepregnancy diabetes mellitus, hypertension, other chronic medical conditions,[2] preeclampsia, placenta previa and prenatal hospital admission.[3] Labour complications shown to increase with advanced maternal age include malpresentation, cephalopelvic disproportion, protraction and arrest disorders, intrapartum decelerations, prolonged second stage labour,[2] operative deliveries[3] and postpartum hemorrhage.

Studies have shown that babies of older mothers are at increased risk for preterm birth, small for gestational age, low one-minute apgar scores and admission to newborn intensive care. Some recent evidence suggests, however, that older women with prudent health behaviours (e.g., smoking abstinence) who receive good quality obstetric care are not at increased risk for complications such as preterm birth and small for gestational age.[2,4]

Rates of live births to older mothers were calculated using vital statistics data.

The proportion of women who are delaying childbearing to later years has increased markedly in Canada in recent years. There is some evidence that this may be associated with adverse outcomes to both mother and infant.

Results

- The live birth rate among older mothers increased steadily between 1981 and 1997. Among women aged 30-34 years, the rate increased from 66.9 per 1,000 in 1981 to 84.9 per 1,000 in 1997 (Figure 1.10). Similarly, increases in rates were observed for older age groups (for example, for women aged 40-44 years, the rate increased from 3.2 in 1981 to 5.3 per 1,000 in 1997) (Figure 1.11).

- The proportion of live births to older mothers has also been steadily increasing over the past 17 years. In 1997, 30.2% of all live births in Canada were to women aged 30-34 years, while women aged 35-39 years accounted for 12.4%, and women 40 years and older accounted for 1.9%. In 1981, these percentages were 18.8%, 4.3%, and 0.6%, respectively (Figure 1.12).

FIGURE 1.10 **Age-specific live birth rate, females 30-39 years,**
Canada (excluding Newfoundland), 1981-1997*

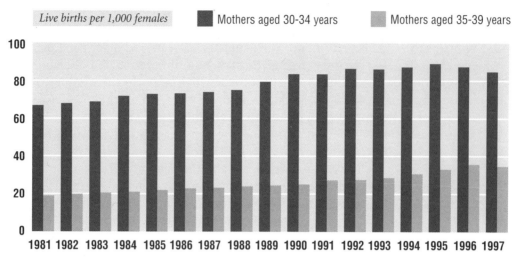

Source: Statistics Canada. Canadian Vital Statistics System, 1981-1997.
* Newfoundland is excluded because data are not available nationally prior to 1991.

FIGURE 1.11 **Age-specific live birth rate, females 40-49 years,**
Canada (excluding Newfoundland), 1981-1997*

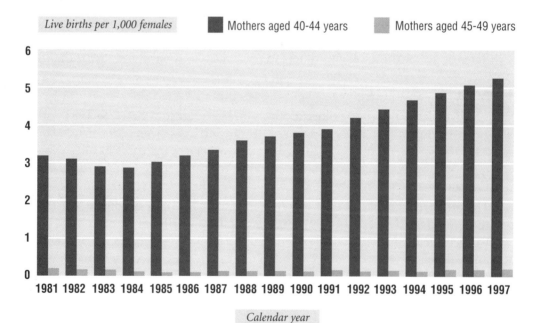

Source: Statistics Canada. Canadian Vital Statistics System, 1981-1997.
* Newfoundland is excluded because data are not available nationally prior to 1991.

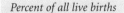

FIGURE 1.12 **Percent of live births to older mothers (≥ 30 years),**
Canada (excluding Newfoundland),* 1981-1997

Percent of all live births

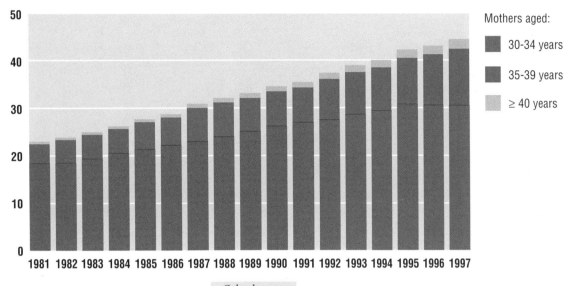

Mothers aged:
- 30-34 years
- 35-39 years
- ≥ 40 years

Calendar year

Source: Statistics Canada. Canadian Vital Statistics System, 1981-1997.

* Newfoundland is excluded because data are not available nationally prior to 1991.

Data Limitations

Canadian data on maternal age are obtained from birth certificates and are unstated in a small fraction of records. Late registered births, stillbirths, ectopic pregnancies and pregnancies that end in abortion are not included in the above statistics.

References

1. Hook EB. Rates of chromosomal abnormalities at different maternal ages. *Obstet Gynecol* 1981; 58: 282-5.

2. Berkowitz GS, Skovron ML, Lapinski RH, Berkowitz RL. Delayed childbearing and the outcome of pregnancy. *N Engl J Med* 1990; 322: 659-64.

3. Leyland AH, Boddy FA. Maternal age and outcome of pregnancy. *N Engl J Med* 1990; 323: 413-4.

4. Prysak M, Lorenz RP, Kisly A. Pregnancy outcome in nulliparous women 35 years and older. *Obstet Gynecol* 1995; 85: 65-70.

Health Services

Labour Induction Rate

The labour induction rate is defined as the number of delivering women whose labour was induced by medical or surgical means (prior to the onset of labour) expressed as a proportion of all delivering women (in a given place and time).

Induction is an obstetric intervention associated with potential risks to both mother and fetus, including neonatal immaturity, uterine hyperstimulation, and prolonged labour.[1] In certain situations, the risks of continuing pregnancy for either mother or fetus will outweigh the risks associated with induction. Indications for labour induction include placental insufficiency (intrauterine growth restriction (IUGR)), poorly-controlled diabetes, insulin-requiring diabetes, prolonged rupture of membranes, postdatism, severe pre-eclampsia and renal failure.[1]

Labour induction rates were estimated using hospitalization data. Ideally, induction rates would include both medical and surgical methods of induction. However, the data presented are limited to medical induction for the following reasons: it is difficult to distinguish between induction and augmentation when considering surgical methods, only a small proportion of all inductions are completed with surgical methods alone, and some jurisdictions only record medical methods in their data.

Labour induction rates varied substantially among Canadian provinces and territories, from a low of 10.4% in the Northwest Territories to a high of 22.1% in Alberta.

Results

- In 1997, the labour induction rate was 18.5% in Canada. This rate is based on cases with a Canadian Classification of Diagnostic, Therapeutic and Surgical Procedures (CCP) code of medical induction and is consistent with the rate of 10%-25% previously estimated by the Society of Obstetricians and Gynaecologists of Canada (SOGC).[2]

- Labour induction rates varied substantially among Canadian provinces and territories, from a low of 10.4% in the Northwest Territories to a high of 22.1% in Alberta (Figure 2.1). These regional differences may be due in part to variations in clinical practice.

FIGURE 2.1 **Labour induction rate, by province/territory,**
Canada (excluding Québec), 1997-1998*

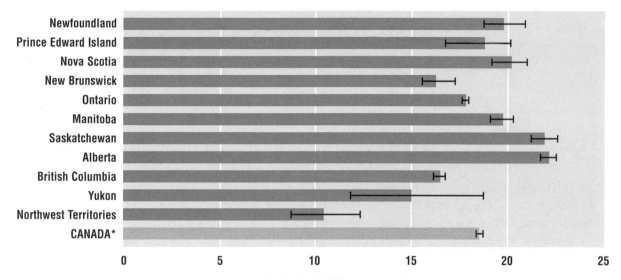

Inductions (95% CI) per 100 hospital deliveries

Sources: Canadian Institute for Health Information. Discharge Abstract Database, 1997-1998.
Manitoba Health, Epidemiology Unit. Perinatal Surveillance Database, 1997-1998.
* Québec data are not included in the Discharge Abstract Database (DAD).
CI — confidence interval.

Data Limitations

Limitations in identifying the proportion of delivering women with induced labour relate to errors in identifying whether the labour was induced or whether existing labour was augmented. Augmentation is defined as the use of medical or surgical means to enhance labour that has already begun spontaneously.

References

1. Keirse MJNC, Chalmers I. Methods of inducing labor. In: Chalmers I, Enkin M, Keirse MJNC (Eds.), *Effective Care in Pregnancy and Childbirth.* Oxford: Oxford University Press, 1989.

2. Society of Obstetricians and Gynaecologists of Canada. *Induction of Labour, SOGC Clinical Practice Guidelines for Obstetrics, Number 23.* Ottawa: SOGC, 1996.

Cesarean Section Rate

The cesarean section (CS) rate is defined as the number of deliveries by CS expressed as a percentage of the total number of deliveries (in a given place and time). The primary CS rate is the number of cesarean deliveries to women who have not previously had a cesarean delivery expressed as a percentage of all deliveries to women who have not had a cesarean delivery previously. This rate includes primiparas (i.e., women giving birth for the first time) and multiparas (i.e., women who have given birth one or more times previously) who have not had a cesarean delivery previously. The repeat CS rate is the number of cesarean deliveries to women who have had a cesarean delivery previously expressed as a percentage of all deliveries to women who have had a previous cesarean delivery.

The proportion of women delivered by CS increased from approximately 5% to nearly 20% in Canada and the United States between the late 1960s and the early 1980s.[1] In Canada today, nearly 20% of births are cesarean births.[2] While this seemingly high rate continues to be of concern because of the potentially increased risks to the mother and the additional costs and lengths of hospital stay associated with cesarean delivery, the rate has remained at the same level — 18% to 19% — for approximately 15 years in spite of efforts to lower it.[2,3] The main strategies to lower the CS rate in Canada have been the establishment of clinical guidelines for CS and efforts to encourage women who have had a previous cesarean delivery to attempt a vaginal delivery (or "VBAC," vaginal birth after cesarean).[4-9]

CS rates were estimated using hospitalization data.

Results

- Between 1994 and 1997, the CS rate increased from 17.8% to 19.1% (Table 2.1). This increase is due to an increase in the primary CS rate, which was more pronounced among women 25 years and older than among younger women (Figure 2.2).

- Primiparous women are more likely to require cesarean delivery than women having their second or third birth who have not had a cesarean delivery previously. Data from Statistics Canada for 1994 to 1997 indicate an increase in the percentage of first births among women aged 25-34 years and 35 years and older (Table 2.2). The percentage of first births to women less than 25 years old did not increase during the same period. Slight increases in the percentage of first births to women in the two older age groups is a possible explanation for the larger increase in the primary CS rate in these two age groups.

- The proportion of women who have had a previous cesarean delivery increased from 9.3% to 10.0% between 1994 and 1997 (Table 2.1). This may be a function of an increasing tendency to record previous cesarean delivery on hospital discharge abstracts rather than a real increase in the proportion of women who have had a previous cesarean delivery. The rate of repeat cesareans decreased somewhat during this time period. Recent efforts to increase the rate of VBAC, as a primary strategy to reduce the rate of cesarean delivery, may have contributed to this trend.

Between 1994 and 1997, the CS rate increased from 17.8% to 19.1%. This increase is due to an increase in the primary CS rate, which was more pronounced among women 25 years and older than among younger women.

Table 2.1 **Cesarean section (CS) rate and percent of women who have had a previous CS,** *Canada (excluding Québec, Nova Scotia and Manitoba),* 1994-1995 to 1997-1998*

Year	CS per 100 hospital deliveries	Primary CS per 100 hospital deliveries	Percent of women with a previous CS**	Percent of CS among women with a previous CS
1994-1995	17.8	12.6	9.3	68.6
1995-1996	18.0	12.8	9.7	66.5
1996-1997	18.6	13.4	9.9	66.5
1997-1998	19.1	13.8	10.0	66.8

Source: Canadian Institute for Health Information. Discharge Abstract Database, 1994-1995 to 1997-1998.

* Québec data are not included in the Discharge Abstract Database (DAD). Nova Scotia and Manitoba are excluded because complete data for all years are not available in the DAD.

** The observed increase over time in the percent of women with previous cesarean delivery may be due to an increased tendency to record previous cesarean delivery in the hospital discharge abstract.

Table 2.2 **Percent of births that were first births, by maternal age,** *Canada, 1994-1997*

	Mother's age		
Year	< 25	25-34	≥ 35
1994	63.5	38.3	24.7
1995	63.7	38.6	25.0
1996	63.5	38.9	25.5
1997	63.1	39.3	25.6

Source: Statistics Canada. Canadian Vital Statistics System, 1994-1997.

FIGURE 2.2 **Primary cesarean section (CS) rate, by maternal age,** *Canada (excluding Québec, Nova Scotia and Manitoba),* 1994-1995 to 1997-1998*

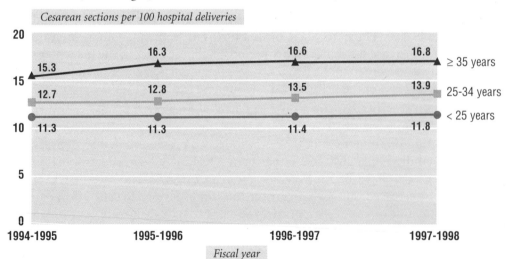

Source: Canadian Institute for Health Information. Discharge Abstract Database, 1994-1995 to 1997-1998.

* Québec data are not included in the DAD. Nova Scotia and Manitoba are excluded because complete data for all years are not available in the DAD.

Data Limitations

Because women having their first baby (particularly women having their first baby at a later age) are at increased risk of cesarean delivery, and because of a continuing trend for women to delay first births, it is preferable to adjust for both of these factors when considering trends over time. Adjustment for both age of mother and parity could not be made, as the latter is not recorded in the DAD.

Another possible limitation is that the denominator used in the calculation of the above CS rates includes hospital deliveries only. While the number of births that occur outside of hospital is small, temporal variation in this number could contribute to variation in CS rates, though any effect is likely small.

Calculation of primary and repeat CS rates using the DAD is not possible before 1994, as the database did not identify vaginal deliveries after cesarean prior to 1994.

References

1.   Notzon FC, Placek PJ, Taffel SM. Comparisons of national cesarean-section rates. *N Engl J Med* 1987; 316: 386-9.

2.   Millar WJ, Nair C, Wadhera S. Declining cesarean section rates: a continuing trend? *Health Rep* 1996; 8: 17-24.

3.   Nair, C. Trends in cesarean deliveries in Canada. *Health Rep* 1991; 3: 203-19.

4.   Helewa M. Cesarean sections in Canada: what constitutes an appropriate rate? *J Soc Obstet Gynaecol Can* 1995; 17: 237-46.

5.   Society of Obstetricians and Gynaecologists of Canada. *Dystocia. Society of Obstetricians and Gynaecologists of Canada Policy Statement.* Ottawa: SOGC, 1995.

6.   Society of Obstetricians and Gynaecologists of Canada. *Vaginal Birth after a Previous Cesarean. Society of Obstetricians and Gynaecologists of Canada Policy Statement.* Ottawa: SOGC, 1993.

7.   Society of Obstetricians and Gynaecologists of Canada. *The Canadian Consensus Conference on Breech Management at Term. Society of Obstetricians and Gynaecologists of Canada Policy Statement.* Ottawa: SOGC, 1994.

8.   Society of Obstetricians and Gynaecologists of Canada. *Fetal Health Surveillance in Labour, Parts 1 through 4. Society of Obstetricians and Gynaecologists of Canada Policy Statement.* Ottawa: SOGC, 1995.

9.   Society of Obstetricians and Gynaecologists of Canada. *Fetal Health Surveillance in Labour, Conclusion. Society of Obstetricians and Gynaecologists of Canada Policy Statement.* Ottawa: SOGC, 1996.

Rate of Operative Vaginal Deliveries

Operative vaginal delivery rates varied considerably among Canadian provinces and territories in 1997.

The rate of operative vaginal deliveries is defined as the number of vaginal births assisted by means of forceps or vacuum extraction expressed as a proportion of all vaginal births (in a given place and time).

Appropriate use of operative vaginal delivery leads to potential benefits for the mother and baby; inappropriate or improper use, however, can be harmful. The choice of forceps or vacuum extraction has been based largely on tradition and training.[1,2] There is a tendency in North America to shift from forceps to vacuum extraction because results from randomized trials have shown that vacuum extraction causes less trauma to mothers and infants.[2,3] However, these randomized trials were too small to assess rare and important outcomes such as intracranial hemorrhage and mortality in infants. There is a need to monitor infant outcomes following forceps and vacuum extractions in routine practice.

Rates of operative vaginal deliveries were estimated using hospitalization data.

Results

- In 1997 in Canada, the overall rate of operative vaginal deliveries was 17.2%. The rate of forceps use was 7.4% and the rate of vacuum extraction was 10.5%. Deliveries in which both forceps and vacuum extraction were used account for the discrepancy between the overall rate and the sum of the individual forceps use and vacuum extraction rates.

- Operative vaginal delivery rates varied considerably among Canadian provinces and territories in 1997 (Figures 2.3, 2.4, 2.5). These regional differences may be due in part to variations in clinical practice.

FIGURE 2.3 **Rate of operative vaginal deliveries, by province/territory,** *Canada (excluding Québec),* * 1997-1998*

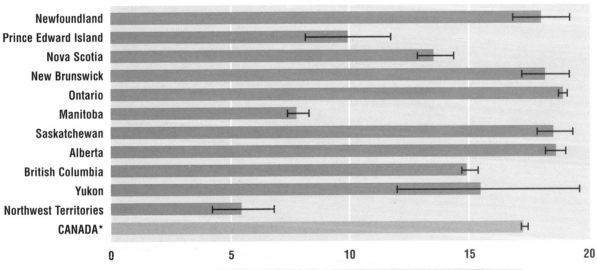

Operative vaginal deliveries (95% CI) per 100 hospital vaginal deliveries

Sources: Canadian Institute for Health Information. Discharge Abstract Database, 1997-1998.
Manitoba Health, Epidemiology Unit. Perinatal Surveillance Database, 1997-1998.

* Québec data are not included in the Discharge Abstract Database (DAD).

CI — confidence interval.

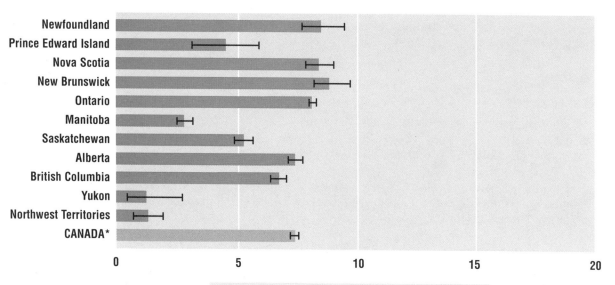

FIGURE 2.4 **Rate of vaginal deliveries by forceps, by province/territory,** *Canada (excluding Québec),* 1997-1998*

Forceps use (95% CI) per 100 hospital vaginal deliveries

Sources: Canadian Institute for Health Information. Discharge Abstract Database, 1997-1998.
Manitoba Health, Epidemiology Unit. Perinatal Surveillance Database, 1997-1998.
* Québec data are not included in the DAD.
CI — confidence interval.

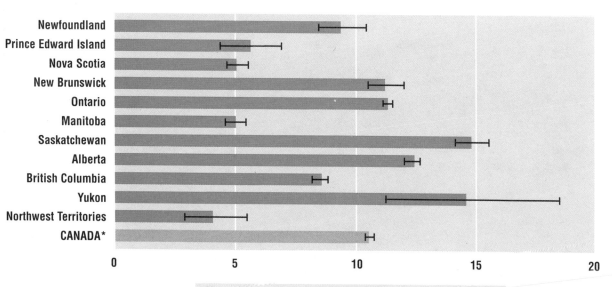

FIGURE 2.5 **Rate of vaginal deliveries by vacuum extraction, by province/territory,** *Canada (excluding Québec),* 1997-1998*

Vacuum extractions (95% CI) per 100 hospital vaginal deliveries

Sources: Canadian Institute for Health Information. Discharge Abstract Database, 1997-1998.
Manitoba Health, Epidemiology Unit. Perinatal Surveillance Database, 1997-1998.
* Québec data are not included in the DAD.
CI — confidence interval.

Data Limitations

Operative vaginal delivery rates were calculated from hospital discharge data. Since instrumental deliveries are considered minor procedures, coding of these procedures may not be as complete as coding for major procedures (e.g., cesarean delivery).

References

1.   Editorial. Vacuum versus forceps. *Lancet* 1984; i: 144.

2.   Johanson RB. Vacuum extraction versus forceps delivery. In: Enkin M, Keirse M, Renfrew M, Neilson J (Eds.), The Cochrane Collaboration: Pregnancy and Childbirth Database, 1994, Disk Issue I.

3.   Johanson RB, Rice C, Doyle M, Arthur J, Anyanwu L, Ibrahim J et al. A randomised prospective study comparing the new vacuum extractor policy with forceps delivery. *Br J Obstet Gynaecol* 1993; 100: 524-30.

Rate of Trauma to the Perineum

The rate of trauma to the perineum is defined as the number of women who had an episiotomy or a delivery resulting in a first-, second-, third- or fourth-degree laceration (tear) of the perineum expressed as a proportion of all women who had a vaginal delivery (in a given place and time).

Episiotomy is one of the most common surgical procedures in Western medicine, yet there is no evidence to support its liberal or routine use.[1,2] Spontaneous lacerations of the perineum range from minor lacerations that do not require repair with sutures to fourth-degree tears which extend through the rectal mucosa to expose the lumen of the rectum. Higher rates of trauma are consistently observed in first vaginal births and with instrumental delivery.[3] Perineal trauma can result in short-term morbidity, such as pain and hemorrhage. Potential long-term morbidity includes protracted pain and difficulties in bowel, urinary and sexual function.[3]

Rates of trauma to the perineum were estimated using hospitalization data.

Results

- In 1997, the Canadian episiotomy rate was 25.4 per 100 vaginal births. The decreasing episiotomy rate in Canada between 1989 and 1997 (Figure 2.6) is due to changes in obstetric practice. These changes may reflect a response to research which demonstrated that the routine use of episiotomy is not justified.

- Increasing laceration rates over the same time period may be a result of a decreased use of episiotomies and/or an increased reporting of lacerations. The increase in lacerations is for first- and second-degree lacerations (Figure 2.6). It is noteworthy that the decline in use of episiotomy has not been accompanied by an increase in the more serious third- and fourth-degree lacerations.

- The 1997 provincial/territorial episiotomy rates ranged from 6.0 per 100 vaginal births in the Yukon to 35.1 per 100 vaginal births in Prince Edward Island (Figure 2.7). These regional differences may be due in part to variations in clinical practice.

The decreasing episiotomy rate in Canada between 1989 and 1997 is due to changes in obstetric practice.

Data Limitations

An important limitation in the surveillance of trauma to the perineum in Canada is the variation that exists in the classification and case definition of perineal trauma. For example, spontaneous lacerations which are minor and do not require suturing may not be enumerated.[3] Alternatively, greater attention to the occurrence of lacerations due to decreasing use of episiotomies may result in increased reporting of less serious lacerations. As well, under-reporting of episiotomies may occur as a result of collection and coding practices.[1]

FIGURE 2.6 Trauma to the perineum by episiotomy and perineal laceration rates, *Canada,* * *1989-1990 to 1997-1998*

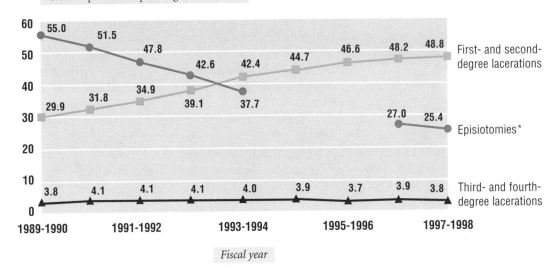

Trauma per 100 hospital vaginal deliveries

First- and second-degree lacerations

Episiotomies*

Third- and fourth-degree lacerations

Fiscal year

Sources: Canadian Institute for Health Information. Discharge Abstract Database, 1989-1990 to 1997-1998.
        Graham et al., 1997.[1]

* 1996-1997 and 1997-1998 episiotomy data and all laceration data exclude Nova Scotia, Québec and Manitoba.
  There were no available episiotomy data for 1994-1995 or 1995-1996.

FIGURE 2.7 Episiotomy rate, by province/territory,
Canada (excluding Québec), * *1997-1998*

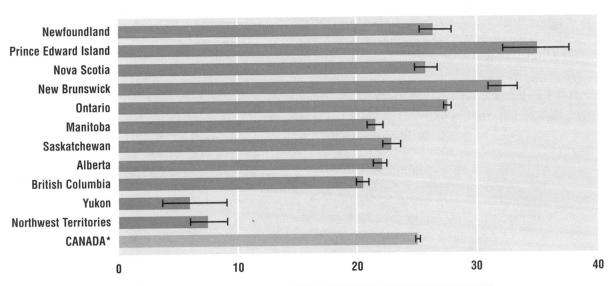

Episiotomies (95% CI) per 100 hospital vaginal deliveries

Sources: Canadian Institute for Health Information. Discharge Abstract Database, 1997-1998.
        Manitoba Health, Epidemiology Unit. Perinatal Surveillance Database, 1997-1998.

* Québec data are not available in the Discharge Abstract Database (DAD).

CI — confidence interval.

References

1. Graham ID, Fowler-Graham D. Episiotomy counts: Trends and prevalence in Canada, 1981/1982 to 1993/1994. *Birth* 1997; 24: 141-7.

2. Argentine Episiotomy Trial Collaborative Group. Routine vs selective episiotomy: A randomised controlled trial. *Lancet* 1993; 342: 1517-8.

3. Renfrew MJ, Hannah W, Albers L, Floyd E. Practices that minimize trauma to the genital tract in childbirth: A systematic review of the literature. *Birth* 1998; 25: 143-60.

Rate of Early Maternal Discharge from Hospital after Childbirth

Between 1989 and 1997, the average maternal length of hospital stay for childbirth declined significantly from 4.0 to 2.3 days for vaginal births and from 6.7 to 4.5 days for cesarean births.

The rate of early maternal discharge from hospital after childbirth is defined as the number of women discharged from hospital early (within two days after vaginal birth or within four days after cesarean birth) expressed as a proportion of all women discharged from hospital after childbirth (in a given place and time).

Early maternal discharge is associated with the quality, efficiency and accessibility of hospital services for childbirth. The length of time that mothers should stay in hospital for childbirth remains controversial. Early postpartum discharge may pose risks to the health of mothers and their infants.[1-3] However, most studies evaluating early postpartum discharge in terms of major maternal outcomes have not yet established significant adverse effects on mothers.[1,4]

Rates of early maternal discharge were estimated using hospitalization data. Results are presented separately for vaginal and cesarean births.

Results

- Between 1989 and 1997, the proportion of mothers who stayed in hospital for less than two days for a vaginal birth showed a marked increase from 3.2% to 25.6% (Figure 2.8). Similarly, the proportion of mothers who stayed in hospital for less than four days for a cesarean birth increased from 2.1% to 31.3%.
- Between 1989 and 1997, the average maternal length of hospital stay for childbirth declined significantly from 4.0 to 2.3 days for vaginal births and from 6.7 to 4.5 days for cesarean births (Table 2.3).
- In 1997, women in Alberta were discharged from hospital following childbirth sooner than women in any other province or territory (Table 2.4, Figure 2.9).

FIGURE 2.8 **Rate of short maternal length of stay (LOS) in hospital for childbirth,** *Canada (excluding Québec, Nova Scotia and Manitoba),* 1989-1990 to 1997-1998*

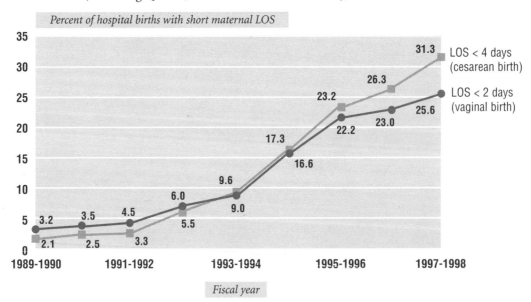

Source: Canadian Institute for Health Information. Discharge Abstract Database, 1989-1990 to 1997-1998.

* Québec data are not included in the Discharge Abstract Database (DAD). Nova Scotia and Manitoba are excluded because complete data for all years are not available in the DAD.

Table 2.3 **Average maternal length of stay (LOS) in hospital for childbirth,** *Canada (excluding Québec, Nova Scotia and Manitoba),* 1989-1990 to 1997-1998*

Year	Mean LOS in days (SD)	
	Vaginal delivery	Cesarean delivery
1989-1990	4.0 (2.0)	6.7 (2.8)
1990-1991	3.8 (1.9)	6.4 (2.8)
1991-1992	3.5 (1.9)	6.2 (2.7)
1992-1993	3.2 (1.8)	5.8 (2.7)
1993-1994	2.9 (1.6)	5.4 (2.6)
1994-1995	2.6 (1.6)	5.0 (2.5)
1995-1996	2.4 (1.6)	4.7 (2.5)
1996-1997	2.3 (1.5)	4.6 (2.4)
1997-1998	2.3 (1.5)	4.5 (2.4)

Source: Canadian Institute for Health Information. Discharge Abstract Database, 1989-1990 to 1997-1998.

* Québec data are not included in the DAD. Nova Scotia and Manitoba are excluded because complete data for all years are not available in the DAD.

SD — standard deviation.

Table 2.4 **Average maternal length of stay (LOS) in hospital for childbirth, by province/territory,** *Canada (excluding Québec),* 1997-1998*

Province/Territory	Mean LOS in days (SD)	
	Vaginal delivery	Cesarean delivery
Newfoundland	3.6 (2.3)	5.5 (3.2)
Prince Edward Island	3.2 (1.7)	5.6 (2.1)
Nova Scotia	2.9 (2.0)	4.8 (3.0)
New Brunswick	2.9 (1.5)	4.8 (2.6)
Ontario	2.1 (1.3)	4.4 (2.3)
Manitoba	2.7 (1.6)	5.1 (2.9)
Saskatchewan	3.0 (1.7)	4.9 (2.6)
Alberta	2.0 (1.4)	4.2 (2.5)
British Columbia	2.5 (1.6)	4.5 (2.5)
Yukon	3.2 (1.9)	4.5 (2.1)
Northwest Territories	2.6 (1.7)	4.8 (1.8)
CANADA*	**2.3 (1.5)**	**4.5 (2.5)**

Sources: Canadian Institute for Health Information. Discharge Abstract Database, 1997-1998.
Manitoba Health, Epidemiology Unit. Perinatal Surveillance Database, 1997-1998.

* Québec data are not included in the DAD.

SD — standard deviation.

FIGURE 2.9 **Rate of short maternal length of stay (LOS) in hospital for childbirth, by province/territory,** *Canada (excluding Québec),* 1997-1998*

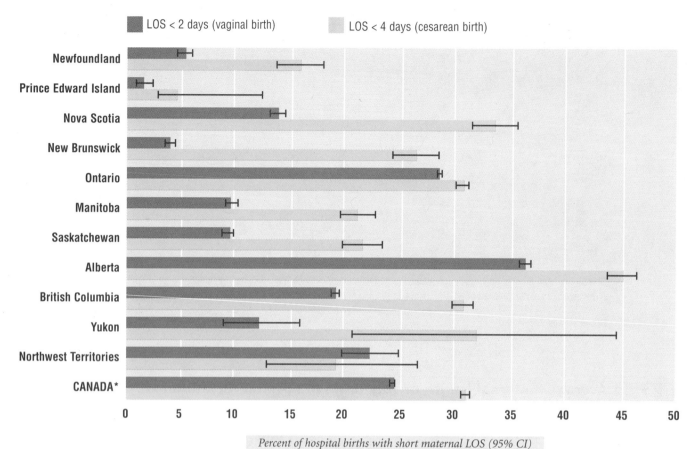

■ LOS < 2 days (vaginal birth)   ■ LOS < 4 days (cesarean birth)

Percent of hospital births with short maternal LOS (95% CI)

Sources: Canadian Institute for Health Information. Discharge Abstract Database, 1997-1998.
Manitoba Health, Epidemiology Unit. Perinatal Surveillance Database, 1997-1998.
* Québec data are not included in the DAD.
CI — confidence interval.

Data Limitations

Information regarding the time of birth is not available on the mother's file in the DAD. As a result, the maternal length of hospital stay reported includes the time between admission and childbirth.

References

1. Dalby DM, Williams JI, Hodnett E, Rush J. Postpartum safety and satisfaction following early discharge. *Can J Public Health* 1996; 87: 90-4.

2. Gloor JE, Kissoon N, Joubert GI. Appropriateness of hospitalization in a Canadian pediatric hospital. *Pediatrics* 1993; 91: 70-4.

3. Wen SW, Liu S, Marcoux S, Fowler D. Trends and variations in length of hospital stay for childbirth in Canada. *Can Med Assoc J* 1998; 158: 875-80.

4. Meikle SF, Lyons E, Hulac P, Orleans M. Rehospitalizations and outpatient contacts of mothers and neonates after hospital discharge after vaginal delivery. *Am J Obstet Gynecol* 1998; 179: 166-71.

Rate of Early Neonatal Discharge from Hospital after Birth

The rate of early neonatal discharge from hospital after birth is defined as the number of newborns discharged from hospital early (within 24 or 48 hours of birth) expressed as a proportion of all newborns discharged from hospital after birth (in a given place and time).

Appropriate early discharge of newborns, taking into account their health status, may increase the efficiency of hospital services and provide other benefits to newborns and their families.[1] However, the question of how long a newborn should stay in hospital after birth remains controversial. Potential risks and benefits of newborn early discharge policies have not been adequately examined by randomized clinical trials. [1-3]

Rates of early neonatal discharge were estimated using hospitalization data. Results are presented separately for low birth weight (1,000-2,499 g) and normal birth weight (≥ 2,500 g) babies.[4]

The rate of early discharge of newborns weighing ≥ 2,500 g increased from 3.1% in 1989 to 28.7% in 1997.

Results

- Between 1989 and 1997, the proportion of newborns weighing 1,000-2,499 g who stayed in hospital for less than two days after birth varied, peaking at 15.0% in 1995 (Figure 2.10). The rate of early discharge of newborns weighing ≥ 2,500 g increased from 3.1% in 1989 to 28.7% in 1997.

FIGURE 2.10 **Rate of early neonatal discharge from hospital after birth,**
Canada (excluding Québec, Nova Scotia and Manitoba), 1989-1990 to 1997-1998*

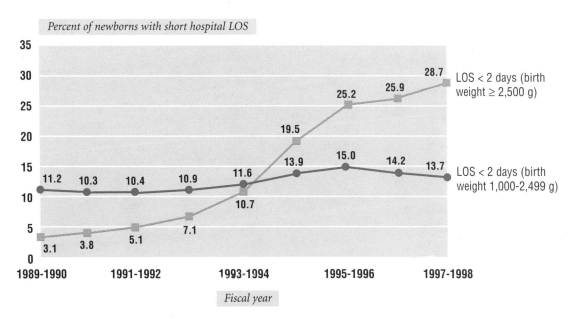

Source: Canadian Institute for Health Information. Discharge Abstract Database, 1989-1990 to 1997-1998.
* Québec data are not included in the Discharge Abstract Database (DAD). Nova Scotia and Manitoba are excluded because complete data for all years are not available in the DAD.
LOS — length of stay.

- For newborns weighing 1,000-2,499 g at birth, the average length of hospital stay at birth decreased from 9.0 days in 1989 to 7.7 days in 1995, and then increased to 7.9 days in 1997 (Table 2.5). For newborns weighing ≥ 2,500 g, the average length of hospital stay after birth decreased steadily, from 3.9 days in 1989 to 2.4 days in 1997.

- In 1997, the Yukon and Northwest Territories had the shortest average neonatal length of stay (LOS) for low birth weight newborns (1,000-2,499 g). However, Alberta had the shortest average LOS for normal birth weight babies (≥ 2,500 g) (Table 2.6). The Northwest Territories had the largest proportion of low birth weight newborns discharged within two days, while Alberta had the largest proportion of normal birth weight newborns discharged within two days (Figure 2.11).

FIGURE 2.11 **Rate of early neonatal discharge from hospital after birth, by province/territory,** *Canada (excluding Québec),* 1997-1998*

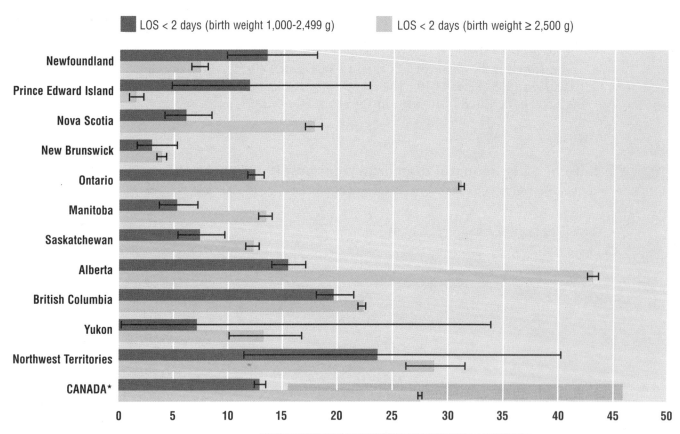

Percent of newborns with short hospital LOS (95% CI)

Sources: Canadian Institute for Health Information. Discharge Abstract Database, 1997-1998.
Manitoba Health, Epidemiology Unit. Perinatal Surveillance Database, 1997-1998.
* Québec data are not included in the DAD.
LOS — length of stay.
CI — confidence interval.

Table 2.5 **Average neonatal length of stay (LOS) in hospital after birth,**
Canada (excluding Québec, Nova Scotia and Manitoba), 1989-1990 to 1997-1998*

Year	Mean LOS in days (SD)	
	Birth weight 1,000-2,499 g	Birth weight ≥ 2,500 g
1989-1990	9.0 (6.7)	3.9 (1.8)
1990-1991	8.9 (6.7)	3.7 (1.8)
1991-1992	8.5 (6.6)	3.5 (1.8)
1992-1993	8.2 (6.7)	3.2 (1.7)
1993-1994	8.1 (6.8)	2.9 (1.7)
1994-1995	7.8 (6.8)	2.6 (1.6)
1995-1996	7.7 (6.8)	2.5 (1.6)
1996-1997	7.8 (6.8)	2.4 (1.6)
1997-1998	7.9 (6.8)	2.4 (1.6)

Source: Canadian Institute for Health Information. Discharge Abstract Database, 1989-1990 to 1997-1998.

* Québec data are not included in the DAD. Nova Scotia and Manitoba are excluded because complete data for all years are not available in the DAD.

SD — standard deviation.

Table 2.6 **Average neonatal length of stay (LOS) in hospital after birth, by province/territory,** *Canada (excluding Québec),* 1997-1998*

Province/ Territory	Mean LOS in days (SD)	
	Birth weight 1,000-2,499 g	Birth weight ≥ 2,500 g
Newfoundland	8.3 (6.8)	3.1 (1.6)
Prince Edward Island	9.6 (7.3)	3.4 (1.8)
Nova Scotia	11.1 (7.3)	2.7 (1.8)
New Brunswick	11.0 (7.2)	3.1 (1.8)
Ontario	7.9 (6.7)	2.3 (1.6)
Manitoba	10.5 (7.2)	2.7 (1.8)
Saskatchewan	9.6 (7.1)	2.9 (1.7)
Alberta	7.7 (6.8)	2.0 (1.6)
British Columbia	7.0 (6.4)	2.5 (1.6)
Yukon	5.1 (2.8)	2.9 (1.7)
Northwest Territories	5.3 (5.3)	2.4 (1.6)
CANADA*	**7.9 (6.8)**	**2.4 (1.6)**

Sources: Canadian Institute for Health Information. Discharge Abstract Database, 1997-1998.
Manitoba Health, Epidemiology Unit. Perinatal Surveillance Database, 1997-1998.

* Québec data are not included in the DAD.

SD — standard deviation.

Data Limitations

In the DAD the hour of birth is not recorded. Therefore it is not possible to obtain the exact duration of hospital stay which is of interest, especially among infants discharged on the first day of life. Ideally, analyses should also be stratified by gestational age at birth; however the DAD does not include information on gestational age.

References

1. Braverman P, Egerter S, Pearl M, Marchi K, Miller C. Problems associated with early discharge of newborn infants. Early discharge of newborns and mothers: a critical review of the literature. *Pediatrics* 1995; 96: 716-26.

2. Lee KS, Perlman M, Ballantyne M, Elliott I, To T. Association between duration of neonatal hospital stay and readmission rate. *J Pediatr* 1995; 127: 758-66.

3. Liu LL, Clemens CJ, Shay DK, Davis RL, Novack AH. The safety of newborn early discharge. The Washington State experience. *J Am Med Assoc* 1997; 278: 293-8.

4. Wen SW, Liu S, Fowler D. Trends and variations in neonatal length of in-hospital stay in Canada. *Can J Public Health* 1998; 89: 115-9.

B

Maternal, Fetal and Infant Health Outcomes

Maternal Health Outcomes

Maternal Mortality Ratio

The maternal mortality ratio (MMR) is defined as the number of maternal deaths per 100,000 live births (in a given place and time).

A country's maternal mortality ratio is considered an important indicator of the general health of the population, the availability and quality of medical care, as well as the status of women.[1] At approximately four maternal deaths reported for every 100,000 live births, Canada has one of the lowest maternal mortality ratios in the world, reflecting our universal access to high quality medical care, our healthy population, and the generally favourable economic and social status of Canadian women.

Statistics Canada reports all deaths annually by age, province/territory and underlying cause. In Canada, up until January 1, 2000, underlying causes of death were classified according to the Ninth Revision of the International Classification of Diseases (ICD-9).[2] Maternal deaths are those where the underlying cause of death has been assigned a numerical code between 630 and 676 under Chapter 11 (Complications of Pregnancy, Childbirth and the Puerperium) of ICD-9.

The definition of maternal death under ICD-9 is:

The death of a woman while pregnant or within 42 days of the termination of the pregnancy, irrespective of the duration and the site of the pregnancy, from any cause related to or aggravated by the pregnancy or its management but not from accidental or incidental causes.

Maternal deaths are considered to be either:

a. Direct obstetric deaths — that is, deaths resulting from obstetric complications of the pregnant state (pregnancy, labour and puerperium); from interventions, omissions or incorrect treatment; or from a chain of events resulting from any of the above; or

b. Indirect obstetric deaths — that is, deaths resulting from previous existing disease or disease that developed during pregnancy, which were not due to direct obstetric causes but were aggravated by the physiologic effects of pregnancy. A definition of "indirect obstetric death" first appeared in the Ninth Revision of the ICD system; deaths considered to be indirect obstetric deaths have, therefore, been included in counts of maternal deaths in Canada only since ICD-9 was adopted for use in this country in 1979.

MMRs were calculated using vital statistics data.

Canada has one of the lowest maternal mortality ratios in the world, reflecting our universal access to high quality medical care, our healthy population, and the generally favourable economic and social status of Canadian women.

Results

- The MMR decreased from 8.2 per 100,000 live births in 1973-1977 to 3.8 per 100,000 live births in 1988-1992 (Figure 3.1). The decline was most pronounced between 1973 and 1982. Although few maternal deaths attributable to indirect causes were reported between 1973 and 1997, a slight increase in the number of these deaths between 1988 and 1997 led to the observed increase in the total MMR for these years. The MMR that includes deaths from direct obstetric causes has decreased consistently since 1973.

- The most common causes of maternal death in Canada are all direct obstetric causes — hypertensive disorders of pregnancy, pulmonary embolism, hemorrhage and ectopic pregnancy (Table 3.1). While maternal deaths from most causes have decreased between the 1970s and 1990s, deaths associated with ectopic pregnancy and those caused by amniotic fluid and other pulmonary embolisms have increased between these two time periods (Table 3.1).

Table 3.1 **Direct maternal deaths by cause,***
Canada, 1973-1977 and 1993-1997

Cause	Ratio per 1,000,000 live births (number)		% change
	1973-1977	1993-1997	
Ectopic pregnancy	4.1 (7)	4.8 (9)	+17
Other abortive outcomes**	8.7 (15)	1.1 (2)	-87
Antepartum hemorrhage	7.6 (13)	4.8 (9)	-37
Hypertensive disorders	12.8 (22)	9.1 (17)	-29
Other pregnancy complications	3.5 (6)	0.5 (1)	-86
Postpartum hemorrhage	9.3 (16)	2.1 (4)	-77
Delivery trauma	5.2 (9)	1.1 (2)	-79
Other delivery complications	9.9 (17)	2.7 (5)	-73
Puerperal sepsis	4.1 (7)	1.1 (2)	-73
Puerperal phlebitis	3.5 (6)	1.1 (2)	-69
Amniotic fluid embolism	4.1 (7)	5.9 (11)	+44
Other pulmonary embolism	2.3 (4)	2.7 (5)	+17
Cerebrovascular disorders	4.1 (7)	3.2 (6)	-22
Other puerperal disorders	2.9 (5)	0.0 (0)	-100
Total direct obstetric deaths	**82.2 (141)**	**40.2 (75)**	**-51**

Source: See references 3-10 at the end of this section.
*Note that the denominator used in this table is 1,000,000 live births rather than 100,000 live births as in Figure 3.1.
**Includes: missed abortion, hydatidiform mole, induced and spontaneous abortions.

FIGURE 3.1 **Maternal mortality ratio (MMR),**
Canada, 1973-1997

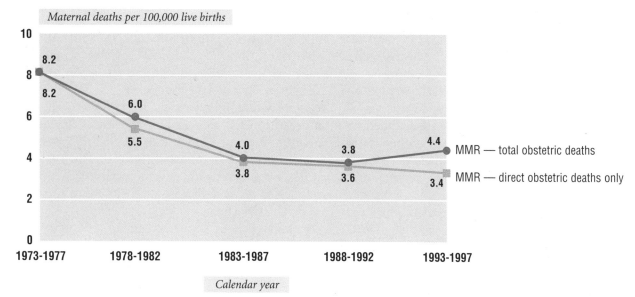

Source: See references 3-10 below.

Data Limitations

Because a number of countries have found that maternal mortality is under-reported by vital records systems, the World Health Organization (WHO) now routinely inflates reported MMRs by a factor of 1.5 to take under-reporting into account when comparing country-specific rates.[1] The Canadian Perinatal Surveillance System (CPSS) is completing a study to determine whether and by how much maternal deaths are under-reported in Canada.

References

1. World Health Organization/UNICEF. *Revised 1990 Estimates of Maternal Mortality: A New Approach by WHO and UNICEF.* Geneva: WHO, 1991.

2. World Health Organization. *Manual of the International Statistical Classification of Diseases, Injuries, and Causes of Death*, 9th Revision. Vol. 1. Geneva: WHO, 1977.

3. Statistics Canada. *Causes of Death, 1973, 1974, 1975, 1976, 1977, 1978, 1979, 1980, 1981, 1982, 1983, 1984, 1985, 1986, 1987.* Ottawa: Statistics Canada, Health Statistics Division (Catalogue No. 84-203-XPB (annual)).

4. Statistics Canada. Causes of Death, 1988. *Health Rep* 1990; (11S): 2(1).

5. Statistics Canada. Causes of Death, 1989. *Health Rep* 1991; (11S): 3(1).

6. Statistics Canada. *Causes of Death, 1990.* Ottawa: Statistics Canada, Health Statistics Division, 1992 (11S): 4(1).

7. Statistics Canada. *Causes of Death, 1991, 1992, 1993, 1994, 1995, 1996, 1997.* Ottawa: Statistics Canada, Health Statistics Division (Catalogue No. 84-208-XPB (annual)).

8. Statistics Canada. Births. *Vital Statistics* 1973; 1.

9. Statistics Canada. *Births and Deaths, 1991, 1992, 1993, 1994, 1995.* Ottawa: Statistics Canada, Health Statistics Division. (Catalogue No. 84-210-XPB (annual)).

10. Statistics Canada. *Births and Deaths 1996, 1997 (shelf tables).* Ottawa: Statistics Canada, Health Statistics Division, 1999 (Catalogue No. 84F0210-XPB (annual)).

Induced Abortion Ratio

The induced abortion ratio is defined as the number of induced abortions per 100 live births (in a given place and time). A related indicator is the age-specific induced abortion rate, defined as the number of induced abortions in a specified age category per 1,000 females in the same age category.

In 1969, a law was passed to regulate abortion under the *Criminal Code*. This law permitted a qualified medical practitioner to perform an abortion, if prior approval was obtained by a Therapeutic Abortion Committee. A 1988 Supreme Court of Canada decision found this process to be unconstitutional. The 1969 law was rendered unenforceable and abortion was effectively decriminalized.[1] Access to abortion services is now viewed as an indicator of society's attitude toward women and their right to reproductive choice.

Induced abortion statistics were obtained from Statistics Canada.[2,3]

Results

In 1997, provincial and territorial induced abortion ratios ranged from 9.5 to 35.5 per 100 live births and the induced abortion rates ranged from 5.0 to 19.2 per 1,000 women of reproductive age.

- In 1997, the induced abortion ratio was 32.9 per 100 live births in Canada. The induced abortion rate was 16.8 per 1,000 females aged 15-44. The induced abortion ratio is increasing at a faster pace than the induced abortion rate, partly due to a decreasing number of live births over time (Figure 3.2).

- In 1997, provincial and territorial induced abortion ratios ranged from 9.5 to 35.5 per 100 live births and the induced abortion rates ranged from 5.0 to 19.2 per 1,000 women of reproductive age. These variations may be attributable to differences in the availability of abortion services, ease of travel to the United States and other local factors[4] (Figure 3.3).

- According to Statistics Canada, women in their twenties accounted for half of all women who obtained an abortion in 1996 and 1997. On average, 28 out of every 1,000 women in their twenties obtained an abortion[3] (Figure 3.4).

Data Limitations

Medically/pharmacologically induced abortions performed in physicians' offices are not systematically reported in abortion statistics. They may become a major under-reporting issue as the use of these procedures increases with time. Additional sources of under-reporting include abortions provided in physicians' offices that have not been designated as abortion facilities, as well as abortions provided to Canadian women in the United States. Age data were missing in 3% of cases. This introduces a small approximation into the calculation of age-specific induced abortion rates.

FIGURE 3.2 **Induced abortion ratio and rate,**
Canada, 1990-1997

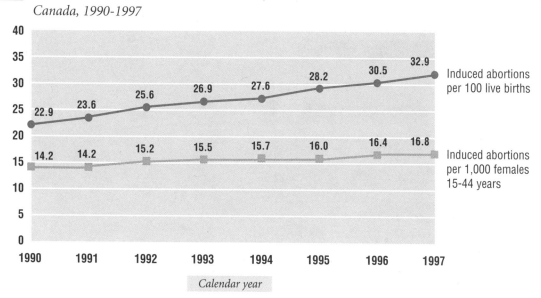

Sources: Statistics Canada. *Therapeutic Abortions, 1995.*
Statistics Canada. Canadian Vital Statistics System, 1990-1997.
Statistics Canada. *The Daily*: Friday, April 7, 2000.
Statistics Canada. Canadian female population estimates, 1990-1997.

FIGURE 3.3 **Induced abortion ratio and rate, by province/territory,** *Canada,* 1997

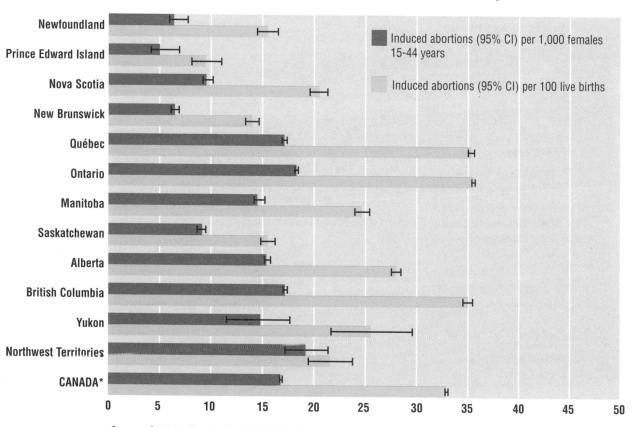

Sources: Statistics Canada. *The Daily*: Friday, April 7, 2000.
Statistics Canada. Canadian Vital Statistics System, 1997.
Statistics Canada. *Births and Deaths, 1997 (shelf tables).*

*Including abortions obtained in the U.S.A. by Canadian women.

CI — confidence interval.

43

FIGURE 3.4 **Age-specific induced abortion rate,**
Canada, 1997

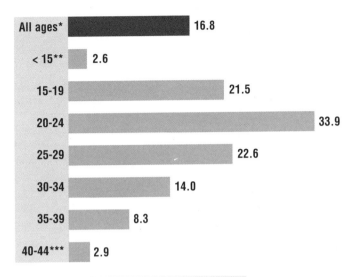

Induced abortions per 1,000 females

Sources: Canadian Institute for Health Information. Therapeutic Abortion Survey, 1997.
Statistics Canada. Health Statistics Division, March 2000.

* Also includes abortions to women over 44. Total includes cases with age not specified (3,547 induced abortions were reported without age specified). Total includes 293 abortions to Canadian women in the U.S.A.

** Rates based on female population aged 14 years.

*** Includes induced abortions to women over 44 years of age at pregnancy termination. Rate based on female population aged 40-44 years.

References

1. Health Canada, Bureau of Reproductive and Child Health. *Induced Abortion Fact Sheet.* April 1998.

2. Statistics Canada. *Therapeutic Abortions, 1995.* Ottawa: Statistics Canada, Health Statistics Division, 1997 (Catalogue No. 82-219-XPB).

3. Statistics Canada. *The Daily:* Friday, April 7, 2000.

4. Statistics Canada. *Statistical Report on the Health of Canadians.* Ottawa: Statistics Canada, 1999 (Catalogue No. 82-570-XPE).

Ectopic Pregnancy Rate

The ectopic pregnancy rate is defined as the number of ectopic pregnancies per 1,000 reported pregnancies (in a given place and time). In this analysis, reported pregnancies include live births, stillbirths, hospital-based induced abortions and ectopic pregnancies. Spontaneous abortions and clinic-based induced abortions are not included in the denominator.

Ectopic pregnancy, defined as the implantation of the blastocyst anywhere other than in the endometrial lining of the uterine cavity,[1] is a significant cause of maternal morbidity and mortality. In industrialized countries, ectopic pregnancy is the leading cause of maternal death during the first trimester of pregnancy, accounting for approximately 10% of all maternal deaths.[2] Some countries have reported an increasing ectopic pregnancy rate; potential explanations for this increase include an increased prevalence of sexually transmitted tubal infections, an increase in the use of contraception that prevents intrauterine but not extra-uterine pregnancies, and better and earlier diagnostic techniques.[1] However, other countries have reported a decrease in the rate of ectopic pregnancies, attributed to declining rates of genital chlamydia.[3]

Ectopic pregnancy rates were estimated using hospitalization data.

In 1997, the ectopic pregnancy rate in Canada was 16.8 per 1,000 reported pregnancies. The rate has been decreasing since 1992.

Results

- In 1997, the ectopic pregnancy rate in Canada was 16.8 per 1,000 reported pregnancies. The rate has been decreasing since 1992 (Figure 3.5).

- The 1997 provincial/territorial ectopic pregnancy rates ranged from 12.2 per 1,000 reported pregnancies in Nova Scotia to 38.0 per 1,000 pregnancies in the Yukon (note the wide confidence intervals for the territories with the highest rates) (Figure 3.6).

- The ectopic pregnancy rate increased with maternal age (Figure 3.7). This is likely due in part to an increased prevalence of scarring of the fallopian tubes among older women.

Data Limitations

An important limitation in the surveillance of ectopic pregnancy in Canada is the reliance on hospital separation data. The availability of risk factor information in hospital records is limited. Also, as pharmacological management of ectopic pregnancy in outpatient settings becomes more common, the enumeration of ectopic pregnancy may be less complete. There may also be variation in the diagnosis of ectopic pregnancy, particularly at very early gestation, and the frequency of subclinical ectopic pregnancy is unknown.[4]

FIGURE 3.5 **Ectopic pregnancy rate,***

*Canada (excluding Québec, Nova Scotia and Manitoba),** 1989-1990 to 1997-1998*

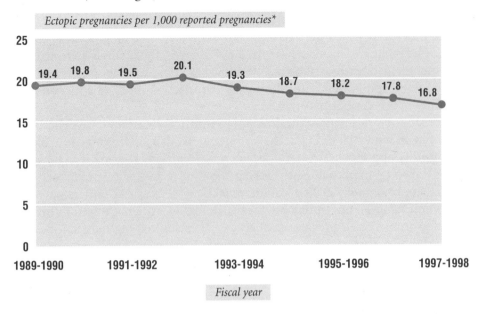

Source: Canadian Institute for Health Information. Discharge Abstract Database, 1989-1990 to 1997-1998.

* Reported pregnancies include live births, stillbirths, hospital-based induced abortions and ectopic pregnancies.

** Québec data are not included in the Discharge Abstract Database (DAD). Nova Scotia and Manitoba are excluded because complete data for all years are not available in the DAD.

FIGURE 3.6 **Ectopic pregnancy rate,* by province/territory,**

*Canada (excluding Québec),** 1997-1998*

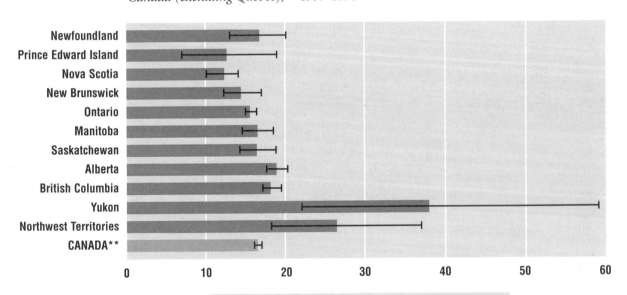

Sources: Canadian Institute for Health Information. Discharge Abstract Database, 1997-1998.
  Manitoba Health, Epidemiology Unit. Perinatal Surveillance Database, 1997-1998.

* Reported pregnancies include live births, stillbirths, hospital-based induced abortions and ectopic pregnancies.

** Québec data are not included in the DAD.

CI — confidence interval.

Maternal Health Outcomes

FIGURE 3.7 **Ectopic pregnancy rate,* by maternal age,**

Canada (excluding Québec),** 1997-1998

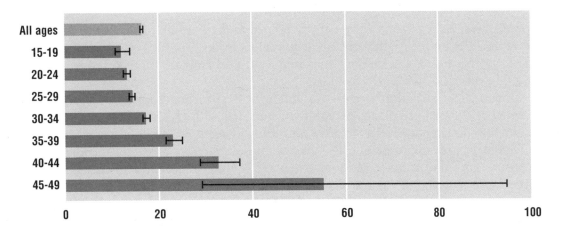

Ectopic pregnancies (95% CI) per 1,000 reported pregnancies*

Sources: Canadian Institute for Health Information. Discharge Abstract Database, 1997-1998.
Manitoba Health, Epidemiology Unit. Perinatal Surveillance Database, 1997-1998.

* Reported pregnancies include live births, stillbirths, hospital-based induced abortions and ectopic pregnancies.

** Québec data are not included in the DAD.

CI — confidence interval.

References

1. Cunningham FG, MacDonald PC, Grant NF, Leveno KJ, Gilstrap LC, Hankins GDV et al. (Eds.). *Williams Obstetrics*, 20th Edition. Stamford, Connecticut: Appleton & Lange, 1997: 607-34.

2. Coste J, Job-Spira N, Fernandez H, Papiernik E, Spira A. Risk-factors for ectopic pregnancy: a case-control study in France, with special focus on infectious factors. *Am J Epidemiol* 1991; 133: 839-49.

3. Egger M, Low N, Smith GD, Lindblom B, Herrmann B. Screening for chlamydial infections and the risk of ectopic pregnancy in a county in Sweden: ecological analysis. *Br Med J* 1998; 316: 1776-80.

4. Orr P, Sherman E, Blanchard J, Fast M, Hammond G, Brunham R. Epidemiology of infection due to *Chlamydia trachomatis* in Manitoba, Canada. *Clin Infect Dis* 1994; 19: 867-83.

Severe Maternal Morbidity Ratio

The severe maternal morbidity ratio is defined as the number of women who experience severe (life-threatening) maternal morbidity per 100,000 live births (in a given place and time). Severe maternal morbidity can also be reported per 100,000 deliveries.

Approximately 15% of direct maternal deaths in Canada are attributed to amniotic fluid embolism. There are no known predisposing risk factors, nor is there understanding of how to prevent this condition.

Because maternal deaths are rare, attention has turned to the question of whether surveillance of health hazards associated with childbearing should include life-threatening events that do not result in death.[1-3] While it has been difficult to quantify the extent of the problem because definitions of life-threatening maternal morbidity and ascertainment methods differ, the Canadian Perinatal Surveillance System (CPSS) has developed a list of conditions associated with pregnancy and childbirth that are potentially life-threatening and that are likely to be captured on hospital discharge summaries. These are: amniotic fluid embolism, obstetrical pulmonary embolism, eclampsia, septic shock, anesthesia complications, cerebrovascular disorders, hemorrhage (antepartum or postpartum) requiring either transfusion or hysterectomy, and rupture of the uterus.

This section highlights amniotic fluid embolism. In future CPSS perinatal health reports, other life-threatening conditions related to pregnancy and childbearing will be discussed.

Amniotic fluid embolism can be defined as the entry of amniotic fluid into maternal blood circulation, resulting in severe disturbance of cardiorespiratory function and coagulopathy.[4] These rare events — with a reported incidence ranging between 1 and 15 per 100,000 deliveries — have been associated with a high case fatality rate (as high as 80%) as well as a high risk of neurological impairment among survivors.[4,5] Approximately 15% of direct maternal deaths in Canada are attributed to amniotic fluid embolism. There are no known predisposing risk factors,[6] nor is there understanding of how to prevent this condition.[7]

Amniotic fluid embolism incidence rates were estimated using hospitalization data.

Results

- Amniotic fluid embolism occurs very rarely in Canada. The overall incidence for the years 1989-1990 through 1997-1998 was 5.6 per 100,000 deliveries (Table 3.2).

- No clear trend is observed in the incidence or case-fatality rate of amniotic fluid embolism over time.

Data Limitations

There is no single criterion upon which a diagnosis of amniotic fluid embolism can be made reliably; definitive diagnoses are made at autopsy.[7] While the accuracy of diagnoses of amniotic fluid embolism cannot be determined with the data source used here, the low case fatality rates suggest that amniotic fluid embolism may be over-reported in the Discharge Abstract Database (DAD). Other diagnoses are known to be mistaken for amniotic fluid embolism.[6] The reported incidence and mortality rates are based on hospital deliveries only. Amniotic fluid embolism may also occur in association with pregnancy termination.

Table 3.2 **Number, recorded incidence and case fatality rate for amniotic fluid embolism,** *Canada (excluding Québec, Nova Scotia and Manitoba),* * *1989-1990 to 1997-1998*

Year	Number of cases	Incidence (per 100,000 deliveries)	Number of deaths	Case fatality rate (per 100 cases)**
1989-1990	10	3.8	2	20.0
1990-1991	17	6.1	1	5.9
1991-1992	12	4.4	1	8.3
1992-1993	22	8.1	3	13.6
1993-1994	12	4.5	2	16.7
1994-1995	8	3.0	1	12.5
1995-1996	17	6.5	3	17.6
1996-1997	17	6.8	5	29.4
1997-1998	18	7.4	1	5.6
Total	**133**	**5.6**	**19**	**14.3**

Source: Canadian Institute for Health Information. Discharge Abstract Database, 1989-1990 to 1997-1998.

* Québec data are not included in the DAD. Nova Scotia and Manitoba are excluded because complete data for all years are not available in the DAD.

** Although the annual number of occurrences and the number of deaths are small, the observed overall case fatality rate of 14.3%, as well as case fatality rates for each year, are low in comparison to case fatality rates of approximately 80% reported in hospital-based studies. This suggests that amniotic fluid embolism may be over-reported in the DAD, perhaps because of a tendency to diagnose less serious events as amniotic fluid embolisms.[5]

Amniotic fluid embolism is one of the indicators that will be assessed in a current quality assurance study of the DAD, which is being carried out by the Canadian Institute for Health Information (CIHI) with the financial support and collaboration of the CPSS.

References

1. Mantel GD, Buchmann E, Rees H, Pattinson RC. Severe acute maternal morbidity: a pilot study of a definition for a near-miss. *Br J Obstet Gynaecol* 1998; 105: 985-90.

2. Baskett TF, Sternadel J. Maternal intensive care and near-miss mortality in obstetrics. *Br J Obstet Gynaecol* 1998; 105: 981-4.

3. Harmer M. Maternal mortality — is it still relevant? *Anesthesia* 1997; 52: 99-100.

4. Morgan M. Amniotic fluid embolism. *Anesthesia* 1979; 34: 20-32.

5. Burrows A, Khoo SK. The amniotic fluid embolism syndrome: 10 years experience at a major teaching hospital. *Aust-N-Z-J Obstet-Gynaecol* 1995; 35: 245-50.

6. Clark SL, Hankins GD, Dudley DA, Dildy GA, Porter TF. Amniotic fluid embolism: analysis of the national registry. *Am J Obstet Gynecol* 1995; 172: 1158-69.

7. Clark SL. New concepts of amniotic fluid embolism: a review. *Obstet-Gynecol-Surv* 1990; 45: 360-8.

Rate of Maternal Readmission after Discharge following Childbirth

Many factors influence maternal readmission rates, including the severity of illness, availability of hospital resources, distance to hospital, hospital admission policies and accessibility of outpatient services.

The maternal hospital readmission rate is defined as the number of mothers readmitted to hospital within three months of initial hospital discharge (following childbirth) expressed as a proportion of the total number of women discharged from hospital following childbirth (in a given place and time).

The maternal readmission rate can serve as a proxy for complications related to childbirth.[1,2] Many factors influence maternal readmission rates, including the severity of illness, availability of hospital resources, distance to hospital, hospital admission policies and accessibility of outpatient services. Generally, maternal readmission following childbirth is an under-researched topic and the impact of maternal readmission on maternal and child health has not been well documented in the scientific literature.[3,4]

Readmission rates were estimated using hospitalization data. Maternal readmission cases were identified by linking obstetric delivery records and readmission records. Results are presented separately for vaginal and cesarean births.

Results

- Between 1990 and 1997, the three-month maternal readmission rate following vaginal birth remained fairly stable, ranging from 2.4% to 2.7% of deliveries. Readmission rates following cesarean births increased, from 3.2% of deliveries in 1990 to 3.9% of deliveries in 1997 (Figure 3.8).

FIGURE 3.8 **Rate of maternal readmission within three months of discharge from hospital following childbirth,***

*Canada (excluding Québec, Nova Scotia and Manitoba),** 1990-1991 to 1997-1998*

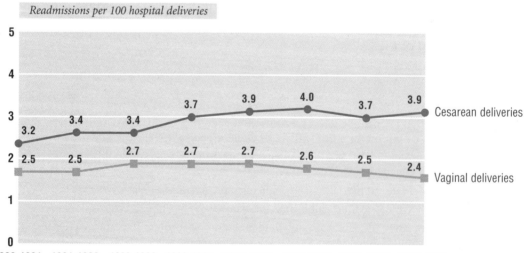

Source: Canadian Institute for Health Information. Discharge Abstract Database, 1990-1991 to 1997-1998.

* Women who were directly transferred to other institutions after childbirth and women with initial length of stay (LOS) > 20 days were excluded from analysis.

** Québec data are not included in the Discharge Abstract Database (DAD). Nova Scotia and Manitoba are excluded because complete data for all years are not available in the DAD.

- In 1995-1997, the three-month maternal readmission rate varied widely by province/territory, both for women with cesarean births and for those with vaginal births (Figure 3.9). These regional differences may be due in part to variations in hospital admission and discharge policies.

- For women who gave birth in hospital between 1995 and 1997, the proportion of readmissions attributable to a given primary diagnosis differed for cesarean vs. vaginal births (Table 3.3).

Data Limitations

Since the identification of maternal readmission is based on record linkage, a few cases of maternal readmission after childbirth would be missed if a link could not be made between the obstetric record and readmission record.

FIGURE 3.9 **Rate of maternal readmission within three months of discharge from hospital following childbirth,* by province/territory,** *Canada (excluding Québec),** 1995-1996 to 1997-1998*

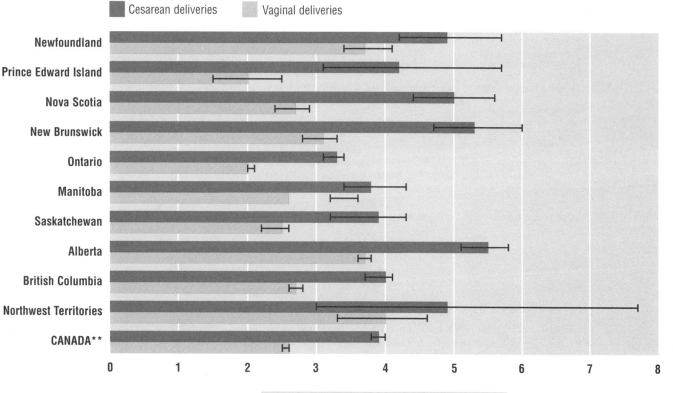

Readmissions (95% CI) per 100 hospital deliveries

Sources: Canadian Institute for Health Information. Discharge Abstract Database, 1995-1996 to 1997-1998.
    Manitoba Health, Epidemiology Unit. Perinatal Surveillance Database, 1995-1996 to 1997-1998.
* Women who were directly transferred after childbirth and women with initial length of stay (LOS) > 20 days were excluded from analysis.
** Québec data are not included in the DAD.
CI — confidence interval.

Canadian Perinatal Health Report, 2000

Table 3.3 **Percent of maternal readmissions within three months of discharge from hospital following childbirth,* by primary diagnosis,** *Canada (excluding Québec),** 1995-1996 to 1997-1998*

Primary diagnosis at readmission (ICD-9 code)	Mode of delivery		
	Total (%)	Cesarean (%)	Vaginal (%)
1. Postpartum hemorrhage (666)	14.4	6.8	17.1
2. Cholelithiasis (574)	13.2	11.4	13.8
3. Major puerperal infection (670)	10.1	10.2	10.1
4. Other and unspecified complications of the puerperium, not elsewhere classified (674)	7.2	20.4	2.6
5. Postpartum care and examination (V24)	3.6	4.4	3.4
6. Persons seeking consultation without complaint of sickness (V65)	3.5	1.5	4.2
7. Infection of the breast and nipple associated with childbirth (675)	3.1	1.9	3.5
8. Other current conditions in the mother classifiable elsewhere, but complicating pregnancy, childbirth or the puerperium (648)	2.2	2.3	2.2
9. Complications of pregnancy, not elsewhere classified (646)	2.3	2.4	2.3
10. Symptoms involving abdomen and pelvis (789)	1.9	1.8	1.9
11. Encounter for contraceptive management (V25)	1.5	0.4	1.9
12. Complications of procedures, not elsewhere classified (998)	1.2	2.4	0.8
13. Venous complications in pregnancy and the puerperium (671)	1.1	1.6	1.0
14. Other diagnoses	34.7	32.6	35.4
Total	**100.0**	**100.0**	**100.0**

Source: Canadian Institute for Health Information. Discharge Abstract Database, 1995-1997.
Manitoba Health, Epidemiology Unit. Perinatal Surveillance Database, 1995-1997.

* Women who were directly transferred after childbirth and women with initial length of stay (LOS) > 20 days were excluded from analysis.

** Québec data are not included in the DAD.

References

1. Meikle SF, Lyons E, Hulac P, Orleans M. Rehospitalizations and outpatient contacts of mothers and neonates after hospital discharge after vaginal delivery. *Am J Obstet Gynecol* 1998; 179: 166-71.

2. Glazener CM, Abdalla M, Stroud P, Naji S, Templeton A, Russell IT. Postnatal maternal morbidity: extent, causes, prevention and treatment. *Br J Obstet Gynaecol* 1995; 102: 282-7.

3. Grimes DA. The morbidity and mortality of pregnancy: still risky business. *Am J Obstet Gynecol* 1994; 170: 1489-94.

4. Danel I, Johnson C, Berg C, Flowers L, Atrash H. Length of maternal hospital stay for uncomplicated deliveries, 1988-1995: The impact of maternal and hospital characteristics. *Matern Child Health J* 1997; 1: 237-42.

Fetal and Infant Health Outcomes

Preterm Birth Rate

The preterm birth rate is defined as the number of live births with a gestational age at birth of less than 37 completed weeks (< 259 days) expressed as a proportion of all live births (in a given place and time).

Preterm birth has been identified as one of the most important perinatal health problems in industrialized nations.[1] Preterm birth accounts for 75%-85% of all perinatal mortality in Canada[2] and is an important determinant of neonatal and infant morbidity, including neurodevelopmental handicap, chronic respiratory problems, infections and ophthalmologic problems.[1] Despite the importance of preterm birth, its etiology and prevention remain poorly understood.

Preterm birth rates were calculated using vital statistics data.

Results

- In 1997, the Canadian preterm birth rate was 7.1 per 100 live births. The preterm birth rate has been increasing since 1981 (Figure 4.1). Potential explanations for this increase include: changes in the frequency and gestational age of multiple-gestation pregnancies, increases in obstetric intervention, greater registration of extremely early-gestation births (20-27 weeks) as live births and increases in the use of ultrasound-based estimates of gestational age.[3,4]

- In 1997, there were markedly higher rates of preterm birth in twins and higher-order births (Figure 4.2). However, singleton births were still responsible for over 80% of all preterm births.

- In 1997, provincial/territorial preterm birth rates ranged from 6.0% in Prince Edward Island to 8.1% in the Northwest Territories (Figure 4.3).

Data Limitations

An important limitation in the surveillance and research of preterm birth is the potential for error in determining gestational age, particularly where menstrual dates are used.[5] This error may be due to inaccurate maternal reporting, the interpretation of post-conception bleeding as normal menses, irregular menstrual cycles or intervening unrecognized pregnancy losses.[1]

Preterm birth accounts for 75%-85% of all perinatal mortality in Canada and is an important determinant of neonatal and infant morbidity, including neuro-developmental handicap, chronic respiratory problems, infections and ophthalmologic problems.

FIGURE 4.1 **Preterm birth rate,**
Canada (excluding Ontario and Newfoundland), 1981-1997*

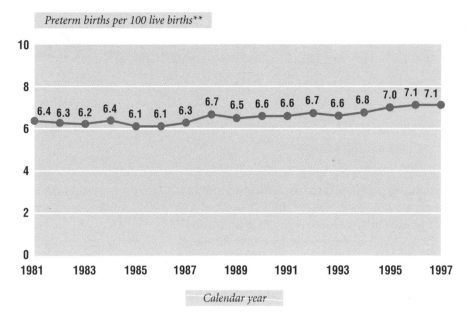

*Preterm births per 100 live births***

Source: Statistics Canada. Canadian Vital Statistics System, 1981-1997.

* Ontario is excluded due to data quality concerns. Newfoundland is excluded because data are not available nationally prior to 1991.

** Excludes live births with unknown gestational age and gestational age < 20 weeks.

FIGURE 4.2 **Preterm birth rates, by single and multiple births,**
Canada (excluding Ontario), 1997*

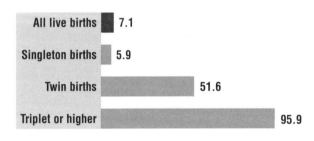

*Preterm births per 100 live births***

Source: Statistics Canada. Canadian Vital Statistics System, 1997.

* Ontario is excluded due to data quality concerns.

** Excludes live births with unknown gestational age and gestational age < 20 weeks.

FIGURE 4.3 **Preterm birth rate, by province/territory,**
Canada (excluding Ontario),* 1997

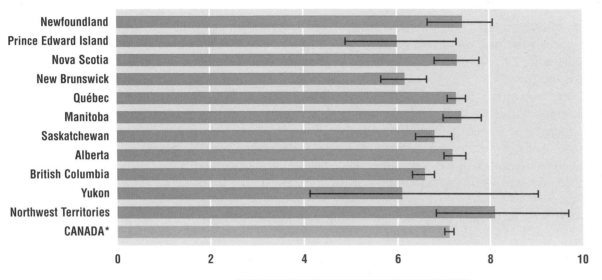

Preterm births (95% CI) per 100 live births**

Source: Statistics Canada. Canadian Vital Statistics System, 1997.

* Ontario is excluded due to data quality concerns.

** Excludes live births with unknown gestational age and gestational age < 20 weeks.

CI — confidence interval.

References

1. Berkowitz GS, Papiernik E. Epidemiology of preterm birth. *Epidemiol Rev* 1993; 15: 414-43.

2. Moutquin JM, Papiernik E. Can we lower the rate of preterm birth? *Bull SOGC* September 1990: 19-20.

3. Joseph KS, Kramer MS, Marcoux S, Ohlsson A, Wen SW, Allen A et al. Determinants of preterm birth rates in Canada from 1981 through 1983 and from 1992 through 1994. *N Engl J Med* 1998; 339: 1434-9.

4. Kramer MS, Platt R, Yang H, Joseph KS, Wen SW, Morin L et al. Secular trends in preterm birth: A hospital-based cohort study. *J Am Med Assoc* 1998; 280: 1849-54.

5. Kramer MS, McLean FH, Boyd ME, Usher RH. The validity of gestational age estimation by menstrual dating in term, preterm, and postterm gestations. *J Am Med Assoc* 1988; 260: 3306-8.

Postterm Birth Rate

Rates of postterm births decreased dramatically in Canada, from 4.3% in 1988 to 1.8% in 1997.

The postterm birth rate is defined as the number of total births (stillbirths and live births) that occur at a gestational age of 42 or more completed weeks (≥ 294 days) of pregnancy expressed as a proportion of total births (in a given place and time).

Postterm birth is associated with increased risk of fetal and infant mortality.[1,2] The main causes for the increased perinatal mortality in postterm births are prolonged labour, unexplained anoxia and neonatal seizures.[3] Controversy exists in the management of postterm pregnancy (intervention versus expectant management). Randomized controlled trials suggest that elective labour induction can reduce perinatal mortality, without an increase in the rates of cesarean deliveries.[4,5]

Postterm birth rates were calculated using vital statistics data.

Results

- Rates of postterm births decreased dramatically in Canada, from 4.3% in 1988 to 1.8% in 1997 (Figure 4.4), caused in part by more frequent use of ultrasound dating, and in part by more frequent labour induction for postterm pregnancies.

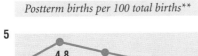

FIGURE 4.4 **Postterm birth rate,**
Canada (excluding Ontario and Newfoundland), 1988-1997*

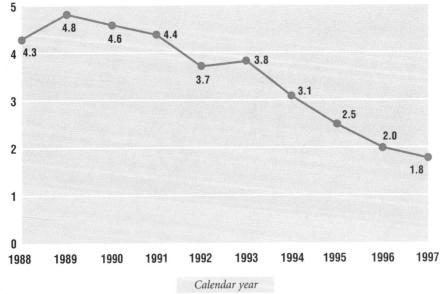

*Posterm births per 100 total births**

Calendar year

Source: Statistics Canada. Canadian Vital Statistics System, 1988-1997.

* Ontario is excluded due to data quality concerns. Newfoundland is excluded because data are not available nationally prior to 1991.

** Excludes live births and stillbirths with unknown gestational age and gestational age < 20 weeks.

- In 1997, rates of postterm birth varied substantially among Canadian provinces and territories, from 0.9% in Newfoundland and Québec to 5.0% in the Yukon (Figure 4.5). These regional variations in postterm births may be due to regional differences in the use of ultrasound dating and/or postterm induction.

FIGURE 4.5 **Postterm birth rate, by province/territory,**
Canada (excluding Ontario), 1997*

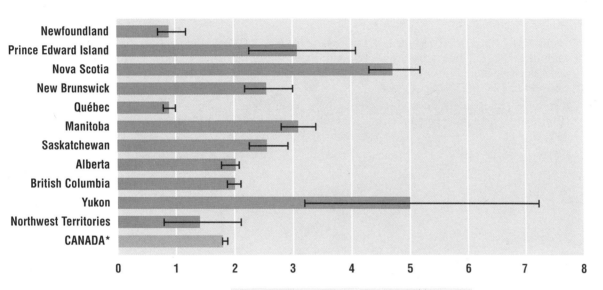

*Postterm births (95% CI) per 100 total births***

Source: Statistics Canada. Canadian Vital Statistics System, 1997.
* Ontario is excluded due to data quality concerns.
** Excludes live births and stillbirths with unknown gestational age and gestational age < 20 weeks.
CI — confidence interval.

Data Limitations

An important limitation in the surveillance and research of postterm birth is the potential for error in determining gestational age, particularly where menstrual dates are used.[6] This error may be due to inaccurate maternal reporting, the interpretation of post-conception bleeding as normal menses, irregular menstrual cycles or intervening unrecognized pregnancy losses.[7]

57

References

1. Hilder L, Costeloe K, Thilaganathan B. Prolonged pregnancy: evaluating gestation-specific risks of fetal and infant mortality. *Br J Obstet Gynaecol* 1998; 105: 169-73.

2. Lucas WE, Anetil AO, Callagan DA. The problem of postterm pregnancy. *Am J Obstet Gynecol* 1965; 91: 241.

3. Naeye RL. Causes of perinatal excess deaths in prolonged gestations. *Am J Epidemiol* 1978; 108: 429-33.

4. Sue-A-Quan AK, Hannah ME, Cohen MM, Foster GA, Liston RM. Effect of labour induction on rates of stillbirth and cesarean section in post-term pregnancies. *Can Med Assoc J* 1999; 160: 1145-9.

5. Hannah ME, Hannah WJ, Hellmann J, Hewson S, Milner R, Willan A, and the Canadian Multicenter Post-Term Pregnancy Trial Group. Induction of labour as compared with serial antenatal monitoring in post-term pregnancy. A randomized controlled trial. *N Engl J Med* 1992; 326: 1587-92.

6. Kramer MS, McLean FH, Boyd ME, Usher RH. The validity of gestational age estimation by menstrual dating in term, preterm, and postterm gestations. *J Am Med Assoc* 1988; 260: 3306-8.

7. Berkowitz GS, Papiernik E. Epidemiology of preterm birth. *Epidemiol Rev* 1993; 15: 414-43.

Fetal Growth: Small-for-Gestational-Age Rate, Large-for-Gestational-Age Rate

1) The small-for-gestational-age (SGA) rate is defined as the number of live births whose birth weights are below the standard 10th percentile of birth weight for gestational age expressed as a proportion of all live births (in a given place and time).

2) The large-for-gestational-age (LGA) rate is defined as the number of live births whose birth weights are above the standard 90th percentile of birth weight for gestational age expressed as a proportion of all live births (in a given place and time).

Alternative cut-offs to determine small for gestational age and large for gestational age can also be used, including the 5th percentile and the 95th percentile of birth weight for gestational age.

Because of the difficulty of in-utero measurement of growth, a cross-sectional measure of fetal growth, birth weight for gestational age, has been used in both clinical and public health practice.[1,2] Fetal growth restriction is associated with increased perinatal morbidity and mortality, whereas accelerated fetal growth can result in macrosomia with associated birth complications.[1] Surveillance of fetal growth indicators can be helpful in identifying populations with high risk of fetal growth restriction and/or macrosomia, and in planning public health programs aimed at reducing risks of fetal growth restriction and macrosomia. In particular, LGA births have been reported to be common among Canadian aboriginal women.[3]

SGA and LGA rates were calculated using vital statistics data. The SGA and LGA cut-offs used for these analyses are based on a standard Canadian population in the mid-1980s.[2]

From 1988-1997, the rate of SGA in Canada decreased. During the same time period the rate of LGA increased.

Results

- From 1988-1997, the rate of SGA in Canada decreased (Figure 4.6). This may be due in part to more frequent use of ultrasound-assisted dating which improves the accuracy of gestational age measurements. During the same time period the rate of LGA increased. In addition to more accurate gestational age measurements, this increase may be due in part to increases in fetal growth over time.

- In 1997, the rate of SGA ranged from 6.2% in the Northwest Territories to 9.9% in the Yukon (Figure 4.7); the rate of LGA ranged from 9.4% in Québec to 15.0% in Prince Edward Island (Figure 4.8). These regional variations in SGA and LGA rates may be caused in part by population profile (i.e., ethnic group) differences. Further research is needed to better understand these trends and variations.

FIGURE 4.6 **Rates of small for gestational age (SGA) and large for gestational age (LGA),**
Canada (excluding Ontario and Newfoundland), 1988-1997*

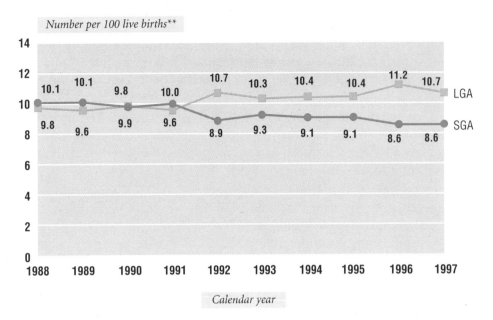

Source: Statistics Canada. Canadian Vital Statistics System, 1988-1997.

* Ontario is excluded due to data quality concerns. Newfoundland is excluded because data are not available nationally prior to 1991.

** Excludes live births with unknown gestational age and birth weight, and gestational age < 20 weeks.

FIGURE 4.7 **Small-for-gestational-age (SGA) rate, by province/territory,**
Canada (excluding Ontario), 1997*

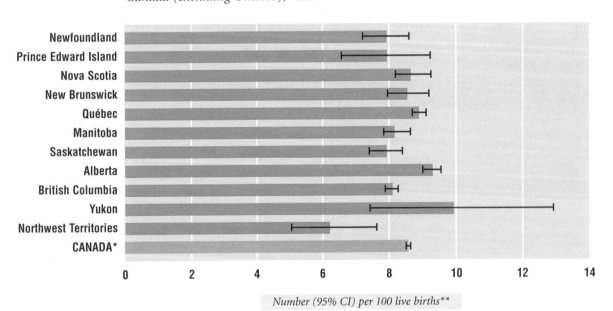

Source: Statistics Canada. Canadian Vital Statistics System, 1997.

* Ontario is excluded due to data quality concerns.

** Excludes live births with unknown gestational age and birth weight, and gestational age < 20 weeks.

CI — confidence interval.

Canadian Perinatal Health Report, 2000

FIGURE 4.8 **Large-for-gestational-age (LGA) rate, by province/territory,**
Canada (excluding Ontario),* 1997

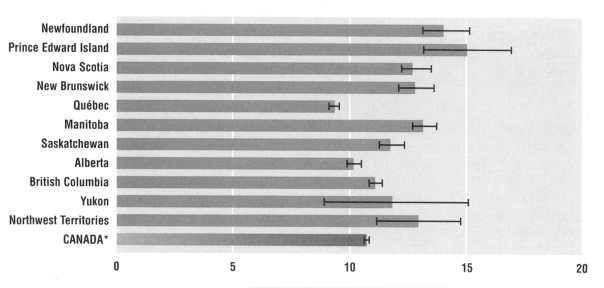

Number (95% CI) per 100 live births**

Source: Statistics Canada. Canadian Vital Statistics System, 1997.
* Ontario is excluded due to data quality concerns.
** Excludes live births with unknown gestational age and birth weight, and gestational age < 20 weeks.
CI — confidence interval.

Data Limitations

An important limitation in the surveillance and research of SGA and LGA birth is the potential for error in determining gestational age, particularly where menstrual dates are used.[4] The accuracy of gestational age estimation can be substantially improved by ultrasound-assisted dating early in the second trimester.[4] SGA and LGA are relative measures, and vary substantially according to the standard used for their calculation. The standard used for this report[2] is now somewhat outdated. A new standard based on better dating information and more sophisticated analytic methods is under development by the Canadian Perinatal Surveillance System (CPSS).

References

1. Cunningham FG, MacDonald PC, Grant NF, Leveno KJ, Gilstrap LC, Hankins GDV et al. (Eds.). *Williams Obstetrics*, 20th Edition. Stamford, Connecticut: Appleton & Lange, 1997.

2. Arbuckle TE, Wilkins R, Sherman GJ. Birth weight percentiles by gestational age in Canada. *Obstet Gynecol* 1993; 81: 39-48.

3. Thomson M. Heavy birthweight in native Indians of British Columbia. *Can J Public Health* 1990; 81: 443-6.

4. Kramer MS, McLean FH, Boyd ME, Usher RH. The validity of gestational age estimation by menstrual dating in term, preterm, and postterm gestations. *J Am Med Assoc* 1988; 260: 3306-8.

Fetal and Infant Mortality Rates

1) The fetal mortality rate is defined as the number of stillbirths ($\geq$ 500 g or $\geq$ 20 weeks of gestation) per 1,000 total births (live births and stillbirths), in a given place and time.

2) The infant mortality rate is defined as the number of deaths of live-born babies in the first year of life per 1,000 live births (in a given place and time).

Fetal mortality can be divided into two components: early fetal deaths (at < 28 completed weeks of gestation) and late fetal deaths (at $\geq$ 28 completed weeks of gestation). Infant mortality can be divided into three components: early neonatal deaths (0-6 days), late neonatal deaths (7-27 days) and postneonatal deaths (28-364 days). Fetal and infant mortality rates can be refined by calculation of birth weight- and age at death-specific mortality rates, and gestational age- and age at death-specific mortality rates. Fetal and infant mortality rates can also be refined by calculation of cause-specific mortality rates. The Canadian Perinatal Surveillance System (CPSS) is currently undertaking a study of temporal trends in cause-specific infant mortality rates.

Infant mortality has been considered the single most comprehensive measure of health in a society. In almost all countries, fetal and infant mortality have decreased dramatically over the last century with improvements in sanitation, nutrition, infant feeding, and maternal and child health care,[1] although the decline has been slower in recent years.[2] Disparities in the risk of infant death remain, however, including in countries such as Canada.

A conceptual framework for perinatal surveillance that focuses on preventable feto-infant mortality was described by Dr. Brian McCarthy, Centers for Disease Control and Prevention, Atlanta, Georgia. Estimates of preventable feto-infant mortality are based on a cross-tabulation of birth weight and age at death that results in a 16-cell table (Table 4.1). Each of the 16 cells represents two aspects of perinatal health: (a) perinatal outcomes (age at death- and birth weight-specific mortality); and (b) determinants of these outcomes (maternal health, maternal care, newborn care and infant environment).

According to this framework, late fetal, neonatal and postneonatal deaths among babies less than 1,500 g may be largely attributable to factors affecting maternal health. Late fetal deaths among babies weighing $\geq$ 1,500 g may result from suboptimal maternal care. Inadequate newborn care including limited access to neonatal intensive care is likely to contribute to early neonatal deaths among babies with birth weights $\geq$ 1,500 g and late neonatal deaths among babies with intermediate birth weight (between 1,500 and 2,499 g). Postneonatal infant deaths among babies with a birth weight of $\geq$ 1,500 g and late neonatal deaths among normal birth weight babies ($\geq$ 2,500 g) are largely attributable to infant environment (e.g., injury prevention and control). Estimates of excess (preventable) feto-infant mortality suggest opportunity gaps among population subgroups in terms of maternal health and the quality of maternal and newborn care, and infant environment. Such information is useful to public health authorities and perinatal health care managers for developing program initiatives.

Fetal and infant mortality rates were calculated using vital statistics data. The calculation of excess (preventable) feto-infant mortality requires a linkage of births and infant deaths, using information from birth and death certificates. Cause-specific mortality has not been included in the current report.

In almost all countries, fetal and infant mortality have decreased dramatically over the last century with improvements in sanitation, nutrition, infant feeding, and maternal and child health care, although the decline has been slower in recent years.

Table 4.1 **Framework for the estimation of preventable feto-infant mortality according to birth weight and age at death**

Birth weight (g)	Late fetal (≥ 28 weeks)	Early neonatal (0-6 days)	Late neonatal (7-27 days)	Postneonatal (28-364 days)
< 1,000	Maternal health			
1,000-1,499				
1,500-2,499	Maternal care	Newborn care		Infant environment
≥ 2,500				

Results

- From 1988 to 1997 the fetal death rate fluctuated between 5.2 and 4.4 per 1,000 total births. The neonatal mortality rate decreased from 4.7 to 3.9 per 1,000 live births and the postneonatal mortality rate decreased from 2.7 to 1.7 per 1,000 neonatal survivors (Figure 4.9).

- In 1997, there were substantial variations in fetal, neonatal and, especially, postneonatal mortality rates among the Canadian provinces and territories (Figures 4.10, 4.11, 4.12).

- In the years 1992-1996, there were opportunities to prevent feto-infant mortality in terms of maternal health, maternal care, neonatal care and infant environment. These opportunities varied substantially according to province/territory. For each province and territory, a rate and a number are provided for maternal health, maternal care, neonatal care and infant environment (Table 4.2). The rate represents the difference between the provincial or territorial rate and the benchmark rate (mortality in births to Québec women with an education of 14 years or more). The number represents the number of excess or fewer (-) deaths in each category, calculated by applying the difference between the provincial/territorial rate and the benchmark to the provincial/territorial population. For example, for Newfoundland in the maternal health category, the fetal, neonatal and postneonatal mortality rate among babies less than 1,500 g is 2.7 per 1,000 births greater than the benchmark, translating into an excess of 85 fetal/infant deaths that could potentially be prevented with interventions in maternal health. For Saskatchewan in the infant environment category, the mortality rate in the late neonatal period among babies ≥ 2,500 g and in the postneonatal period among babies with a birth weight of ≥ 1,500 g is 1.8 per 1,000 births greater than the benchmark, translating into an excess of 127 infant deaths that could potentially be prevented with interventions in infant environment.

- Detailed tabulations of Canadian birth weight-specific and gestational age-specific infant mortality rates for 1994-1996 and interprovincial/territorial variations in birth weight-specific and gestational age-specific infant mortality for the years 1992-1996 are presented in Appendix E.

Estimates of excess (preventable) feto-infant mortality suggest opportunity gaps among population subgroups in terms of maternal health and the quality of maternal and newborn care, and infant environment.

FIGURE 4.9 **Rates of fetal, neonatal and postneonatal deaths,**
Canada (excluding Newfoundland),* 1988-1997

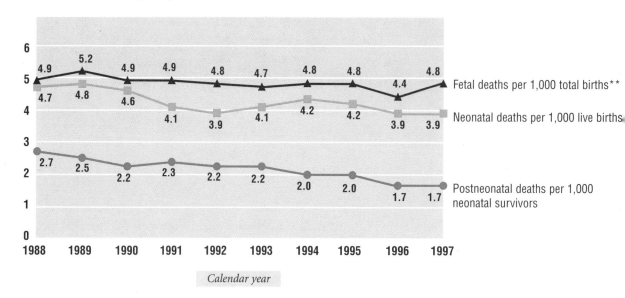

Source: Statistics Canada. Canadian Vital Statistics System, 1988-1997.

* Newfoundland is excluded because data are not available nationally prior to 1991.

** Fetal death rates exclude births with known birth weight of < 500 grams. Ontario is excluded from fetal death rates due to data quality concerns.

FIGURE 4.10 **Fetal death rate,* by province/territory,**
Canada (excluding Ontario),** 1997

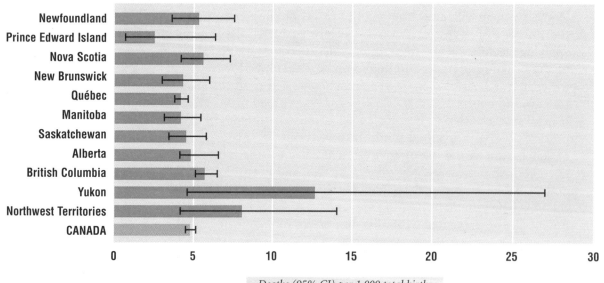

Source: Statistics Canada. Canadian Vital Statistics System, 1997.

*Fetal death rates exclude births with known birth weight of < 500 grams.

** Ontario is excluded due to data quality concerns.

CI — confidence interval.

FIGURE 4.11 **Neonatal death rate, by province/territory,**
Canada, 1997

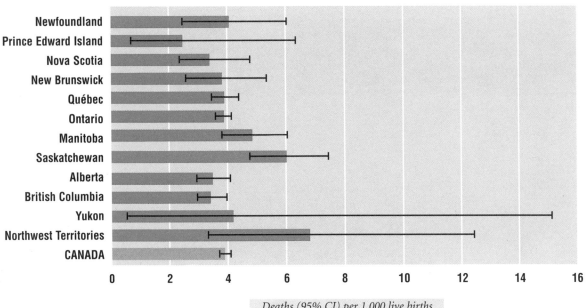

Deaths (95% CI) per 1,000 live births

Source: Statistics Canada. Canadian Vital Statistics System, 1997.
CI — confidence interval.

FIGURE 4.12 **Postneonatal death rate, by province/territory,**
Canada, 1997

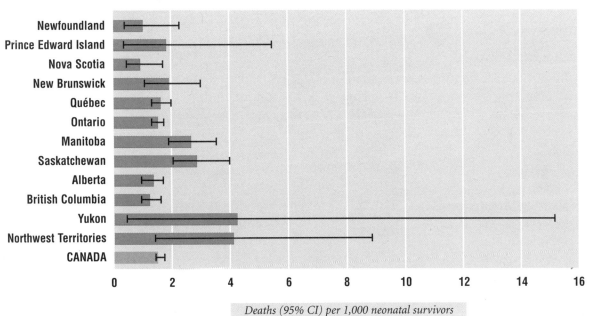

Deaths (95% CI) per 1,000 neonatal survivors

Source: Statistics Canada. Canadian Vital Statistics System, 1997.
CI — confidence interval.

Table 4.2 **Rate (per 1,000 births) of excess feto-infant mortality and number of preventable deaths,* by type of intervention opportunity and province/territory,**

Canada (excluding Ontario),** 1992-1996

| Province/Territory | Intervention opportunity | | | | | | | |
| | Maternal health | | Maternal care | | Neonatal care | | Infant environment | |
	Excess mortality rate	Number of preventable deaths	Excess mortality rate	Number of preventable deaths	Excess mortality rate	Number of preventable deaths	Excess mortality rate	Number of preventable deaths
Newfoundland	2.7	85	0.7	22	0.6	19	0.7	22
Prince Edward Island	1.6	14	2.2	19	0.0	0	0.6	5
Nova Scotia	2.1	118	1.7	96	0.1	6	0.3	17
New Brunswick	1.3	58	1.7	75	0.4	18	0.7	31
Québec	1.1	499	0.7	318	0.1	45	0.3	136
Manitoba	3.9	320	1.5	123	0.2	16	1.2	98
Saskatchewan	2.7	190	1.6	113	0.5	35	1.8	127
Alberta	2.7	540	1.6	320	0.2	40	1.0	200
British Columbia	1.8	420	1.0	233	0.0	0	0.7	163
Yukon	(-0.1)	(-0)	2.9	7	0.0	0	2.3	6
Northwest Territories	2.6	21	2.5	20	0.7	6	6.5	52
CANADA**	**1.9**	**2,129**	**1.1**	**1,317**	**0.1**	**188**	**0.7**	**852**

Source: Statistics Canada. Canadian Vital Statistics System, 1992-1996.

* The benchmark is mortality in births to mothers in the province of Québec with an education of ≥ 14 years (1990-1991 data). In the birth-infant death linked file, all live births at < 22 weeks and < 500 g were assumed to have died on the first day of life and were classified as such.

** Ontario is excluded due to data quality concerns.

Data Limitations

Vital statistics data are subject to registration errors, particularly among extremely small, immature newborns.[3,4] The linkage of births and infant deaths results in 2%-3% of deaths remaining unlinked (this percentage excludes Ontario data).

References

1. Buehler JW, Kleinman JC, Hodgue CJ, Strauss LT, Smith JC. Birth weight-specific infant mortality, United States, 1960 to 1980. *Public Health Rep* 1987; 102: 151-61.

2. Kleinman JC. The slowdown in the infant mortality decline. *Paediatr Perinat Epidemiol* 1990; 4: 373-81.

3. Joseph KS, Kramer MS. Recent trends in Canadian infant mortality rates: Effect of changes in registration of live newborns weighing less than 500 grams. *Can Med Assoc J* 1996; 155: 1047-52.

4. Joseph KS, Allen A, Kramer MS, Cyr M, Fair M for the Fetal-Infant Mortality Study Group of the Canadian Perinatal Surveillance System. Changes in the registration of stillbirths less than 500g in Canada, 1985-95. *Pediatr Perinat Epidemiol* 1999; 13: 278-87.

Severe Neonatal Morbidity Rate

The severe neonatal morbidity rate is defined as the number of infants identified as having severe neonatal morbidity in the first month of life expressed as a proportion of all live born infants (in a given place and time).

Severe morbid conditions during the neonatal period are important predictors of postneonatal morbidity and disability.[1] Classification of the conditions that constitute severe neonatal morbidity may vary. However, certain conditions are more likely to predict long-term disability, including severe respiratory distress syndrome (RDS), sepsis, seizures, severe intraventricular hemorrhage, persistent fetal circulation, and multisystem congenital anomalies. Moreover, these conditions are often associated with each other. For example, intraventricular hemorrhage is predictive of the development of seizures and persistent fetal circulation is linked with sepsis and RDS.

The rate of RDS decreased during the early 1990s, followed by a stable rate in recent years.

This section highlights RDS. In future Canadian Perinatal Surveillance System (CPSS) perinatal health reports, other conditions will be discussed.

Rates of RDS were estimated using hospitalization data.

Results

- In 1997, the rate of RDS was 10.7 per 1,000 live births in Canada. The rate of RDS decreased during the early 1990s, followed by a stable rate in recent years (Figure 4.13).

FIGURE 4.13 **Respiratory distress syndrome (RDS) rate,***
*Canada (excluding Québec, Nova Scotia and Manitoba),** 1989-1990 to 1997-1998*

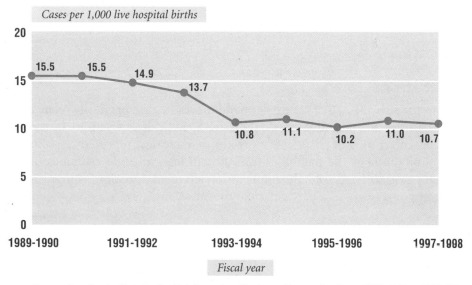

Source: Canadian Institute for Health Information. Discharge Abstract Database, 1989-1990 to 1997-1998.

* RDS cases include infants diagnosed during the birth admission only.

** Québec data are not included in the Discharge Abstract Database (DAD). Nova Scotia and Manitoba are excluded because complete data for all years are not available in the DAD.

- Provincial and territorial rates of RDS varied widely from 2.6 per 1,000 live births in the Northwest Territories to 19.4 per 1,000 live births in Prince Edward Island (Figure 4.14). This wide regional variation in rates may be due in part to differences in the application of the case definition of RDS.

FIGURE 4.14 **Respiratory distress syndrome (RDS) rate,* by province/territory,** *Canada (excluding Québec),** 1997-1998*

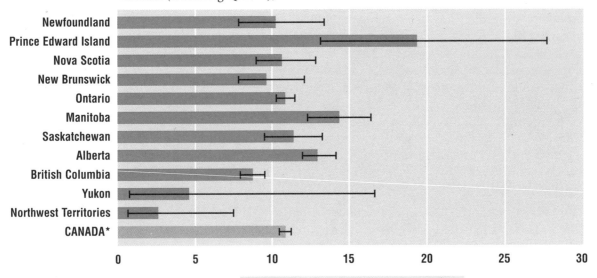

Cases (95% CI) per 1,000 live hospital births

Sources: Canadian Institute for Health Information. Discharge Abstract Database, 1997-1998.
Manitoba Health, Epidemiology Unit. Perinatal Surveillance Database, 1997-1998.
* RDS cases include infants diagnosed during the birth admission only.
** Québec data are not included in the DAD.
CI — confidence interval.

Data Limitations

Limitations in the surveillance of severe neonatal morbidity are primarily related to limitations in the hospital discharge databases. Specifically, variations in the case definitions and coding of particular morbidities may affect reported rates. In general, the limitations of the databases utilized will lead to underestimates of severe neonatal morbidity. As well, the information as coded does not distinguish between degrees of severity of a particular condition.

References

1. Behrman RE, Shiono PH. Neonatal risk factors. In: Fanhroff AA, Martin RJ (Eds.), *Neonatal-Perinatal Medicine. Diseases of the Fetus and Infant,* 6th Edition. Vol. 1. St. Louis: Mosby Publications, 1997: 3-12.

Multiple Birth Rate

The multiple birth rate is defined as the number of live births and stillbirths following a multiple gestation pregnancy expressed as a proportion of all live births and stillbirths (in a given place and time).

Multiple births are at increased risk of being preterm,[1] of intrauterine growth restriction, retinopathy, intraventricular hemorrhage and bronchopulmonary dysplasia.[2] These infants may require additional health care services, including neonatal intensive care.

Multiple birth rates were calculated using vital statistics data.

Results

- Rates of multiple birth increased steadily over time, from 2.1% in 1988 to 2.5% in 1997 (Figure 4.15). An increase in births to older mothers and increased use of fertility treatments and assisted conception are the main reasons for the recent increase in multiple births.[3]

- In 1997, with the exception of the Yukon, rates of multiple birth were similar among Canadian provinces and territories (Figure 4.16). The higher rate in the Yukon must be interpreted with caution, as the rate is based on a small number of births.

An increase in births to older mothers and increased use of fertility treatments and assisted conception are the main reasons for the recent increase in multiple births.

FIGURE 4.15 **Rate of multiple births,**
Canada (excluding Newfoundland), 1988-1997*

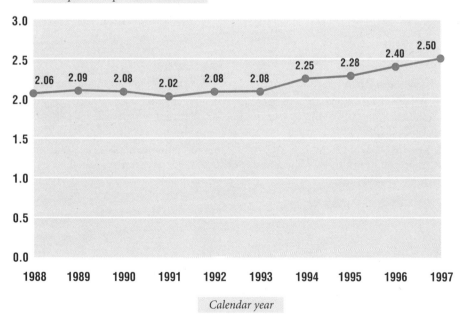

Multiple births per 100 total births

Source: Statistics Canada. Canadian Vital Statistics System, 1988-1997.

* Newfoundland is excluded because data are not available nationally prior to 1991.

69

FIGURE 4.16 **Rate of multiple births, by province/territory,**
Canada, 1997

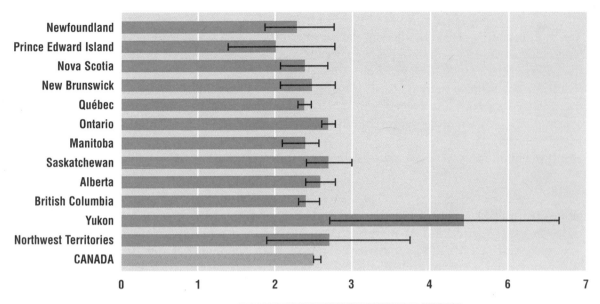

Multiple births (95% CI) per 100 total births

Source: Statistics Canada. Canadian Vital Statistics System, 1997.
CI — confidence interval.

Data Limitations

Canadian data on multiple births are obtained from birth certificates and may be subject to some transcribing errors.

References

1. Newman RB, Ellings JM. Antepartum management of the multiple gestation: the case for specialized care. *Semin Perinatol* 1995; 19: 387-403.

2. Millar WJ, Wadhera S, Nimrod C. Multiple births: trends and patterns in Canada, 1974-1990. *Health Rep* 1992; 4: 223-50.

3. Wilcox LS, Kiely JL, Melvin CL, Martin MC. Assisted reproductive technologies: estimates of their contribution to multiple births and newborn hospital days in the United States. *Fertil Steril* 1996; 65: 361-6.

Prevalence of Congenital Anomalies

The prevalence of congenital anomalies is defined as the number of individual live born or stillborn infants with at least one congenital anomaly expressed as a proportion of the total number of live births and stillbirths (in a given place and time).

Congential anomalies, birth defects and congenital malformations are terms currently used to describe developmental disorders present at birth.[1] Congenital anomalies are a leading cause of all infant deaths and one of the top 10 causes of potential years of life lost.[2] The most prevalent categories of congenital anomalies in Canada are musculoskeletal anomalies, congenital heart defects and central nervous system anomalies, such as neural tube defects (NTDs).

The prevalence of congenital anomalies is estimated using data from the Canadian Congenital Anomalies Surveillance System (CCASS). This report highlights NTDs. The current interest in NTDs lies both in the disability and death they cause, as well as the opportunity to address their occurrence through primary prevention. Furthermore, the evaluation of primary prevention strategies, such as the Canadian policy of fortifying food with folic acid will require careful surveillance of NTD rates over time.

Congenital anomalies are a leading cause of all infant deaths and one of the top 10 causes of potential years of life lost.

Results

- In 1997, the NTD birth prevalence in Canada was 7.6 per 10,000 total births (excludes Québec, as 1997 data for Québec were not available).

- In recent years, the NTD birth prevalence has been decreasing (Figure 4.17), possibly reflecting decreased incidence due to improved nutrition, vitamin supplementation or both. The decreased birth prevalence may also be due to prenatal diagnosis and termination of affected pregnancies.

- In 1997, provincial and territorial NTD birth prevalence ranged from 0.0 to 11.5 per 10,000 births (Figure 4.18). Regional differences in prenatal diagnosis with subsequent termination of affected pregnancies is probably the main reason for variation in regional rates. However, regional differences in the presence of both known and unknown risk factors for NTDs may also exist.

Data Limitations

One of the major limitations in tracking congenital anomalies such as NTDs is the absence of mandatory and standardized national reporting of anomalies that are detected prenatally and result in the termination of the affected pregnancy. Failure to account for these cases results in an underestimate of the true NTD rate and limits interpretation of temporal trends. As well, the availability, completeness and source of data from different regions in Canada have varied over recent years, also limiting the comprehensiveness and consistency of temporal trends.[3]

FIGURE 4.17 **Neural tube defect (NTD) rate,**

Canada (excluding Québec and Nova Scotia), 1989-1997*

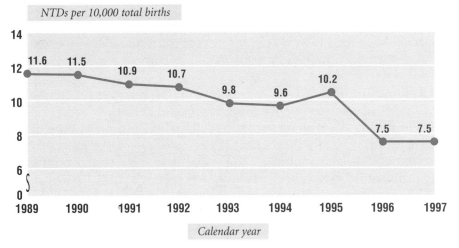

Source: Health Canada. Canadian Congenital Anomalies Surveillance System, 1989-1997.

* Québec and Nova Scotia are excluded because data are not available for all years.

FIGURE 4.18 **Neural tube defect (NTD) rate, by province/territory,**

Canada (excluding Québec), 1997*

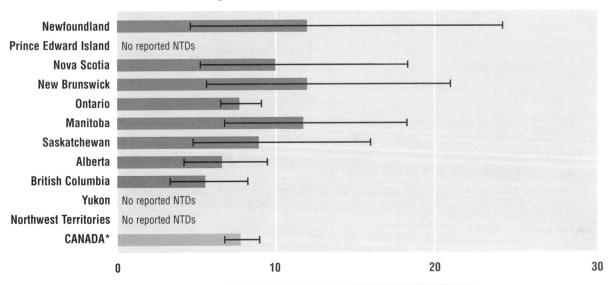

Source: Health Canada. Canadian Congenital Anomalies Surveillance System, 1997.

* Québec is excluded as data for 1997 were not available.

CI — confidence interval.

References

1. Moore KL, Persaud TVN. *Before we are born: essentials of embryology and birth defects.* 5th Edition. Philadelphia: W.B. Saunders Company, 1998.

2. Premature mortality due to congenital anomalies — United States. *MMWR* 1988; 37: 505-6.

3. Health Canada. *Measuring Up.* Ottawa: Minister of Public Works and Government Services Canada, 1999 (Catalogue No. H42-2/82-1999E).

Rate of Neonatal Hospital Readmission after Discharge at Birth

The neonatal hospital readmission rate is defined as the number of newborns who are readmitted to hospital within 28 days of birth expressed as a proportion of all newborns discharged from hospital after birth (in a given place and time). This indicator can also be specified as the rate of readmission within seven days after birth.

Newborn readmission rates have been used as one outcome to evaluate the quality of perinatal health care.[1-3] Newborn readmission rates are related to the length of hospital stay after birth,[4,5] and are one measure of the impact of hospital discharge policies.

Neonatal hospital readmission rates were estimated using hospitalization data. Cases of neonatal readmission were identified by internal record linkage of the Discharge Abstract Database (DAD), which involves matching live birth records to cases of readmission.

Results

- The neonatal hospital readmission rate increased significantly, from 2.8 per 100 live births in 1989 to 4.0 per 100 live births in 1997 (Figure 4.19). Although many factors may contribute to neonatal readmission, the practice of early discharge of newborns without application of guidelines[6] may be related to recently increasing neonatal readmission.

- In 1997, neonatal readmission rates varied widely across Canadian provinces and territories (Figure 4.20). The readmission rate was highest in the Northwest Territories (6.8 per 100 live births) and lowest in Prince Edward Island (1.5 per 100 live births). The provinces and territories with higher neonatal readmission rates also tended to have shorter average length of hospital stay at birth and earlier age at readmission.[7]

- The most common reasons for neonatal readmission were neonatal jaundice, feeding problems, sepsis, dehydration and inadequate weight gain (Figure 4.21). The causes for neonatal readmission changed considerably over time. For example, neonatal jaundice accounted for 21.2% of readmissions in 1989, compared with 38.7% in 1997.

Data Limitations

Concerns with regard to the accuracy and completeness of the record linkage may arise due to newborn transfers and home births. As well, differences in health status at birth, initial length of hospital stay and other issues may confound the association between length of hospital stay at birth and neonatal readmission.

Although many factors may contribute to neonatal readmission, the practice of early discharge of newborns without application of guidelines may be related to recently increasing neonatal readmission.

FIGURE 4.19 **Rate of neonatal hospital readmission after discharge at birth,** *Canada (excluding Québec, Nova Scotia and Manitoba),* 1989-1990 to 1997-1998*

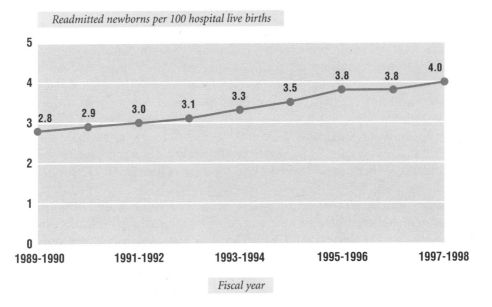

Readmitted newborns per 100 hospital live births

Fiscal year

Source: Canadian Institute for Health Information. Discharge Abstract Database,1989-1990 to 1997-1998.

* Québec data are not included in the DAD. Nova Scotia and Manitoba are excluded because complete data for all years are not available in the DAD.

FIGURE 4.20 **Rate of neonatal hospital readmission after discharge at birth, by province/territory,** *Canada (excluding Québec and Manitoba),* 1997-1998*

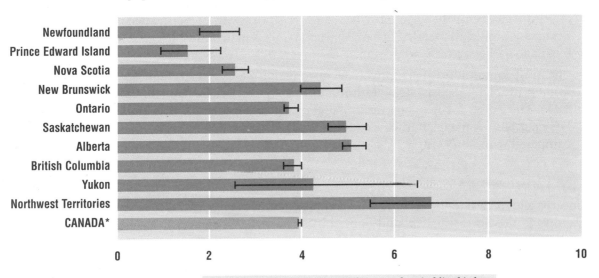

Readmitted newborns (95% CI) per 100 hospital live births

Source: Canadian Institute for Health Information. Discharge Abstract Database, 1997-1998.

* Québec data are not included in the DAD. Complete Manitoba data were not available.

CI — confidence interval.

FIGURE 4.21 **Principal diagnosis for readmitted newborns,**
Canada (excluding Québec, Nova Scotia and Manitoba)*, 1989-1990 and 1997-1998

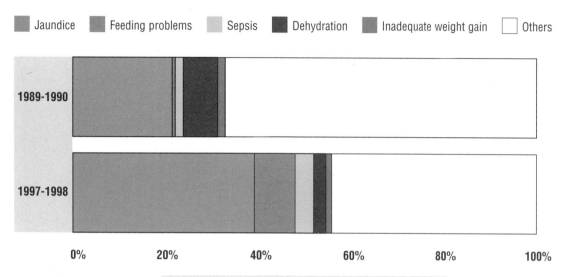

Percentage of readmitted newborns by principal diagnosis

Source: Canadian Institute for Health Information. Discharge Abstract Database, 1989-1990 and 1997-1998.
* Québec data are not included in the DAD. Nova Scotia and Manitoba are excluded because complete data for all years are not available in the DAD.

References

1. Braverman P, Egerter S, Pearl M, Marchi K, Miller C. Problems associated with early discharge of newborn infants. Early discharge of newborns and mothers: a critical review of the literature. *Pediatrics* 1995; 96: 716-26.

2. Liu LL, Clemens CJ, Shay DK, Davis RL, Novack AH. The safety of newborn early discharge. The Washington State experience. *J Am Med Assoc* 1997; 278: 293-8.

3. Britton JR, Britton HL, Beebe SA. Early discharge of the term newborn: a continued dilemma. *Pediatrics* 1994; 94: 291-5.

4. Lee KS, Perlman M, Ballantyne M, Elliott I, To T. Association between duration of neonatal hospital stay and readmission rate. *J Pediatr* 1995; 127: 758-66.

5. Lee KS, Perlman M. The impact of early obstetric discharge on newborn health care. *Curr Opin Pediatr* 1996; 8: 96-101.

6. Canadian Paediatric Society and Society of Obstetricians and Gynaecologists of Canada. Facilitating discharge home following a normal term birth. *Paediatr Child Health* 1996; 1: 165-8.

7. Liu S, Wen SW, McMillan D, Trouton K, Fowler D, McCourt C. Increased neonatal readmission rate associated with decreased length of hospital stay at birth in Canada. *Can J Public Health* 2000; 91: 46-50.

Bibliography

Abel EL (Ed.). *Fetal Alcohol Syndrome, from Mechanism to Prevention.* New York: CRC Press, 1996.

Abel EL. "Moderate" drinking during pregnancy: cause for concern? *Clin Chim Acta* 1996; 246: 149-54.

American Academy of Pediatrics, Work Group on Breastfeeding. Breastfeeding and the use of human milk. *Pediatrics* 1997; 100: 1035-9.

Arbuckle TE, Wilkins R, Sherman GJ. Birth weight percentiles by gestational age in Canada. *Obstet Gynecol* 1993; 81: 39-48.

Argentine Episiotomy Trial Collaborative Group. Routine vs selective episiotomy: A randomised controlled trial. *Lancet* 1993; 342: 1517-8.

Baskett TF, Sternadel J. Maternal intensive care and near-miss mortality in obstetrics. *Br J Obstet Gynaecol* 1998; 105: 981-4.

Behrman RE, Shiono PH. Neonatal risk factors. In: Fanhroff AA, Martin RJ (Eds.), *Neonatal-Perinatal Medicine. Diseases of the Fetus and Infant,* 6th Edition. Vol. 1. St. Louis: Mosby Publications, 1997: 3-12.

Berkowitz GS, Papiernik E. Epidemiology of preterm birth. *Epidemiol Rev* 1993; 15: 414-43.

Berkowitz GS, Skovron ML, Lapinski RH, Berkowitz RL. Delayed childbearing and the outcome of pregnancy. *N Engl J Med* 1990; 322: 659-64.

Braverman P, Egerter S, Pearl M, Marchi K, Miller C. Problems associated with early discharge of newborn infants. Early discharge of newborns and mothers: a critical review of the literature. *Pediatrics* 1995; 96: 716-26.

Breastfeeding Committee for Canada. *Breastfeeding Statement of the Breastfeeding Committee for Canada.* 1996.

Britton JR, Britton HL, Beebe SA. Early discharge of the term newborn: a continued dilemma. *Pediatrics* 1994; 94: 291-5.

Bryan EM. The intrauterine hazards of twins. *Arch Dis Child* 1986; 61: 1044-5.

Buehler JW, Kleinman JC, Hodgue CJ, Strauss LT, Smith JC. Birth weight-specific infant mortality, United States, 1960 to 1980. *Public Health Rep* 1987; 102: 151-61.

Burrows A, Khoo SK. The amniotic fluid embolism syndrome: 10 years experience at a major teaching hospital. *Aust-N-Z-J-Obstet-Gynaecol* 1995; 35: 245-50.

Canadian Centre for Health Information. *Births 1990.* Ottawa: Statistics Canada, 1992 (Catalogue No. 82-003S14).

Canadian Institute for Health Information. Website (www.cihi.ca). Accessed February 7, 2000.

Canadian Paediatric Society, Dieticians of Canada and Health Canada. *Nutrition for Healthy Term Infants.* Ottawa: Minister of Public Works and Government Services Canada, 1998.

Canadian Paediatric Society and Society of Obstetricians and Gynaecologists of Canada. Facilitating discharge home following a normal term birth. *Paediatr Child Health* 1996; 1: 165-8.

Chen J, Fair M, Wilkins R, Cyr M and the Fetal and Infant Mortality Study Group of the Canadian Perinatal Surveillance System. Maternal education and fetal and infant mortality in Quebec. *Health Rep* 1998; 10: 53-64.

Clark SL. New concepts of amniotic fluid embolism: a review. *Obstet-Gynecol-Surv* 1990; 45: 360-8.

Clark SL, Hankins GD, Dudley DA, Dildy GA, Porter TF. Amniotic fluid embolism: analysis of the national registry. *Am J Obstet Gynecol* 1995; 172: 1158-69.

Coste J, Job-Spira N, Fernandez H, Papiernik E, Spira A. Risk-factors for ectopic pregnancy: a case-control study in France, with special focus on infectious factors. A*m J Epidemiol* 1991; 133: 839-49.

Creasy RK, Merkatz IR. Prevention of preterm birth: clinical opinion. *Obstet Gynecol* 1990; 76: 2S-4S.

Crowley P. Interventions for preventing or improving the outcome of delivery at or beyond term (Cochrane Review). In: *The Cochrane Library, Issue 1*. Oxford: Update Software, 2000.

Cunningham FG, MacDonald PC, Grant NF, Leveno KJ, Gilstrap LC, Hankins GDV et al. (Eds.). *Williams Obstetrics*, 20th Edition. Stamford, Connecticut: Appleton & Lange, 1997.

Dalby DM, Williams JI, Hodnett E, Rush J. Postpartum safety and satisfaction following early discharge. *Can J Public Health* 1996; 87: 90-4.

Danel I, Johnson C, Berg C, Flowers L, Atrash H. Length of maternal hospital stay for uncomplicated deliveries, 1988-1995: The impact of maternal and hospital characteristics. *Matern Child Health J* 1997; 1: 237-42.

Dzakpasu S, Joseph KS, Kramer MS, Allen AC. The Matthew Effect: infant mortality in Canada and internationally. *Pediatrics* 2000; 106: e5.

Editorial. Vacuum versus forceps. *Lancet* 1984; i: 144.

Edwards N, Sims-Jones N, Hotz S. *Pre and Postnatal Smoking: A Review of the Literature*. Ottawa: Health Canada, 1996.

Egger M, Low N, Smith GD, Lindblom B, Herrmann B. Screening for chlamydial infections and the risk of ectopic pregnancy in a county in Sweden: ecological analysis. *Br Med J* 1998; 316: 1776-80.

Fair M. The development of national vital statistics in Canada: Part 1 — From 1605 to 1945. *Health Rep* 1994; 6: 355-68.

Fair M, Cyr M. The Canadian Birth Data Base: a new research tool to study reproductive outcomes. *Health Rep* 1993; 5: 281-90.

Fair M, Cyr M, Allen AC, Wen SW, Guyon G, MacDonald RC et al. *Validation Study for a Record Linkage of Births and Infant Deaths in Canada*. Ottawa: Statistics Canada, 1999 (Catalogue No. 84F0013-XIE).

Federal, Provincial and Territorial Advisory Committee on Population Health. *Strategies for Population Health: Investing in the Health of Canadians*. Ottawa: Minister of Supply and Services Canada, 1994.

Final Report of the Royal Commission on Aboriginal Peoples. Ottawa, 1996. (Available: www.inac.gc.ca/ch/rcap/index_e.html).

Fisk NM, Trew G. Two's company, three's a crowd for embryo transfer. *Lancet* 1999; 354: 1572-3.

Fraser AM, Brockert JE, Ward RH. Association of young maternal age with adverse reproductive outcomes. *N Engl J Med* 1995; 332: 1113-7.

Gladstone J, Levy M, Nulman I, Koren G. Characteristics of pregnant women who engage in binge alcohol consumption. *Can Med Assoc J* 1997; 156: 789-94.

Gladstone J, Nulman I, Koren G. Reproductive risks of binge drinking during pregnancy. *Reprod Toxicol* 1996; 10: 3-13.

Glazener CM, Abdalla M, Stroud P, Naji S, Templeton A, Russell IT. Postnatal maternal morbidity: extent, causes, prevention and treatment. *Br J Obstet Gynaecol* 1995; 102: 282-7.

Gloor JE, Kissoon N, Joubert GI. Appropriateness of hospitalization in a Canadian pediatric hospital. *Pediatrics* 1993; 91: 70-4.

Graham ID, Fowler-Graham D. Episiotomy counts: Trends and prevalence in Canada, 1981/1982 to 1993/1994. *Birth* 1997; 24: 141-7.

Grimes DA. The morbidity and mortality of pregnancy: still risky business. *Am J Obstet Gynecol* 1994; 170: 1489-94.

Grobman WA, Peaceman AM. What are the rates and mechanisms of first and second trimester pregnancy loss in twins? *Clin Obstet Gynecol* 1998; 41: 37-45.

Hannah ME, Hannah WJ, Hellmann J, Hewson S, Milner R, Willan A and the Canadian Multicenter Post-Term Pregnancy Trial Group. Induction of labour as compared with serial antenatal monitoring in post-term pregnancy. A randomized controlled trial. *N Engl J Med* 1992; 326: 1587-92.

Harmer M. Maternal mortality — is it still relevant? *Anesthesia* 1997; 52: 99-100.

Health Canada. *Canadian Perinatal Surveillance System Progress Report.* Ottawa: Minister of Supply and Services Canada, 1995.

Health Canada. *Canadian Perinatal Surveillance System Progress Report 1997-1998.* Ottawa: Minister of Public Works and Government Services Canada, 1999.

Health Canada. *Joint Statement: Prevention of Fetal Alcohol Syndrome (FAS), Fetal Alcohol Effects (FAE) in Canada.* Ottawa: Health Canada, October 1996 (Catalogue No. H39-348/1996E).

Health Canada. *Measuring Up.* Ottawa: Minister of Public Works and Government Services Canada, 1999 (Catalogue No. H42-2/82-1999E).

Health Canada. *Perinatal Health Indicators for Canada: A Resource Manual.* Ottawa: Minister of Public Works and Government Services Canada, 2000 (Catalogue No. H49-135/2000E) .

Health Canada, Bureau of Reproductive and Child Health. *Induced Abortion Fact Sheet.* April 1998.

Helewa M. Cesarean sections in Canada: what constitutes an appropriate rate? *J Soc Obstet Gynaecol Can* 1995; 17: 237-46.

Hilder L, Costeloe K, Thilaganathan B. Prolonged pregnancy: evaluating gestation-specific risks of fetal and infant mortality. *Br J Obstet Gynaecol* 1998; 105: 169-73.

Hook EB. Rates of chromosomal abnormalities at different maternal ages. *Obstet Gynecol* 1981; 58: 282-5.

Howell EM, Blondel B. International infant mortality rates: bias from reporting differences. *Am J Public Health* 1994; 84: 850-2.

Huebert K, Rafts C. *Fetal Alcohol Syndrome and Other Alcohol Related Birth Defects,* 2nd Edition. Edmonton: Alberta Alcohol and Drug Abuse Commission, 1996.

Huizinga D, Loeber R, Thornberry TP. Longitudinal study of delinquency, drug use, sexual activity and pregnancy among children and youth in three cities. *Public Health Rep* 1993; 108 (S1): 90-6.

Johanson RB. Vacuum extraction versus forceps delivery. In: Enkin M, Keirse M, Renfrew M, Neilson J (Eds.), The Cochrane Collaboration: Pregnancy and Childbirth Database, 1994, Disk Issue I.

Johanson RB, Rice C, Doyle M, Arthur J, Anyanwu L, Ibrahim J et al. A randomised prospective study comparing the new vacuum extractor policy with forceps delivery. *Br J Obstet Gynaecol* 1993; 100: 524-30.

Joseph KS, Allen A, Kramer MS, Cyr M, Fair M for the Fetal-Infant Mortality Study Group of the Canadian Perinatal Surveillance System. Changes in the registration of stillbirths less than 500g in Canada, 1985-95. *Paediatr Perinat Epidemiol* 1999; 13: 278-87.

Joseph KS, Kramer MS. Recent trends in Canadian infant mortality rates: Effect of changes in registration of live newborns weighing less than 500 grams. *Can Med Assoc J* 1996; 155: 1047-52.

Joseph KS, Kramer MS, Allen AC, Cyr M, Fair M, Ohlsson A et al. for the Fetal-Infant Mortality Study Group of the Canadian Perinatal Surveillance System. Gestational age- and birth weight-specific declines in infant mortality in Canada, 1985-94. *Paediatr Perinat Epidemiol* (in press).

Joseph KS, Kramer MS, Marcoux S, Ohlsson A, Wen SW, Allen A et al. Determinants of preterm birth rates in Canada from 1981 through 1983 and from 1992 through 1994. *N Engl J Med* 1998; 339: 1434-9.

Kallen B. Congenital malformations in twins: a population study. *Acta Genet Med Gemello Roma* 1986; 35: 167-78.

Keirse MJNC, Chalmers I. Methods of inducing labor. In: Chalmers I, Enkin M, Keirse MJNC (Eds.), *Effective Care in Pregnancy and Childbirth.* Oxford: Oxford University Press, 1989.

79

Kleinman JC. The slowdown in the infant mortality decline. *Paediatr Perinat Epidemiol* 1990; 4: 373-81.

Kramer MS, Demissie K, Yang H, Platt RW, Sauve R, Liston R for the Fetal and Infant Health Study Group of the Canadian Perinatal Surveillance System. The contribution of mild and moderate preterm birth to infant mortality. *J Am Med Assoc* 2000; 284: 843-9.

Kramer MS, McLean FH, Boyd ME, Usher RH. The validity of gestational age estimation by menstrual dating in term, preterm, and postterm gestations. *J Am Med Assoc* 1988; 260: 3306-8.

Kramer MS, Platt R, Yang H, Joseph KS, Wen SW, Morin L et al. Secular trends in preterm birth: A hospital-based cohort study. *J Am Med Assoc* 1998; 280: 1849-54.

Lee KS, Perlman M. The impact of early obstetric discharge on newborn health care. *Curr Opin Pediatr* 1996; 8: 96-101.

Lee KS, Perlman M, Ballantyne M, Elliott I, To T. Association between duration of neonatal hospital stay and readmission rate. *J Pediatr* 1995; 127: 758-66.

Leyland AH, Boddy FA. Maternal age and outcome of pregnancy. *N Engl J Med* 1990; 323: 413-4.

Liu LL, Clemens CJ, Shay DK, Davis RL, Novack AH. The safety of newborn early discharge. The Washington State experience. *J Am Med Assoc* 1997; 278: 293-8.

Liu S, Heaman M, Demissie K, Wen SW, Marcoux S, Kramer MS. Association between maternal readmission and obstetric conditions at childbirth: a case-control study. Presented at the 13th Annual Meeting of the Society for Pediatric and Perinatal Epidemiologic Research, Seattle, Washington, June 2000.

Liu S, Heaman M, Kramer MS, Demissie K, Turner L for the Maternal Mortality and Morbidity Study Group of the Canadian Perinatal Surveillance System. Association between length of hospital stay, obstetric conditions at childbirth, and maternal rehospitalization [submitted for publication].

Liu S, Wen SW. Development of record linkage of hospital discharge data for the study of neonatal readmission. *Chron Dis Can* 1999; 20: 77-81.

Liu S, Wen SW, McMillan D, Trouton K, Fowler D, McCourt C. Increased neonatal readmission rate associated with decreased length of hospital stay at birth in Canada. *Can J Public Health* 2000; 91: 46-50.

Lucas WE, Anetil AO, Callagan DA. The problem of postterm pregnancy. *Am J Obstet Gynecol* 1965; 91: 241.

Mantel GD, Buchmann E, Rees H, Pattinson RC. Severe acute maternal morbidity: a pilot study of a definition for a near-miss. *Br J Obstet Gynaecol* 1998; 105: 985-90.

McCarthy B. The risk approach revisited: A critical review of developing country experience and its use in health planning. In: Liljestrand J, Povey WG (Eds.), *Maternal Health Care in an International Perspective. Proceedings of the XXII Berzelius Symposium, 1991 May 27-29, Stockholm, Sweden.* Sweden: Uppsala University, 1992: 107-24.

Meikle SF, Lyons F, Hulac P, Orleans M. Rehospitalizations and outpatient contacts of mothers and neonates after hospital discharge after vaginal delivery. *Am J Obstet Gynecol* 1998; 179: 166-71.

Millar WJ, Nair C, Wadhera S. Declining cesarean section rates: a continuing trend? *Health Rep* 1996; 8: 17-24.

Millar WJ, Wadhera S, Nimrod C. Multiple births: trends and patterns in Canada, 1974-1990. *Health Rep* 1992; 4: 223-50.

Miller HS, Lesser KB, Reed KL. Adolescence and very low birth weight infants: A disproportionate association. *Obstet Gynecol* 1996; 87: 83-8.

Mitchell A. Rising deaths among infants stun scientists. *Globe and Mail* [Toronto]. June 2, 1995: A4.

Monnier A. Les méthodes d'analyse de la mortalité infantile. In: *Manuel d'analyse de la mortalité.* Paris: INED, 1985: 52-5.

Moore KL, Persaud TVN. *Before we are born: essentials of embryology and birth defects.* 5th Edition. Philadelphia: W.B. Saunders Company, 1998.

Morgan M. Amniotic fluid embolism. *Anesthesia* 1979; 34: 20-32.

Morrison JC. Preterm birth: a puzzle worth solving. *Obstet Gynecol* 1990; 76: 5S-12S.

Moutquin JM, Papiernik E. Can we lower the rate of preterm birth? *Bull SOGC* September 1990: 19-20.

Naeye RL. Causes of perinatal excess deaths in prolonged gestations. *Am J Epidemiol* 1978; 108: 429-33.

Nair C. Trends in cesarean deliveries in Canada. *Health Rep* 1991; 3: 203-19.

Newman RB, Ellings JM. Antepartum management of the multiple gestation: the case for specialized care. *Semin Perinatol* 1995; 19: 387-403.

Notzon FC, Placek PJ, Taffel SM. Comparisons of national cesarean-section rates. *N Engl J Med* 1987; 316: 386-9.

Orr P, Sherman E, Blanchard J, Fast M, Hammond G, Brunham R. Epidemiology of infection due to *Chlamydia trachomatis* in Manitoba, Canada. *Clin Infect Dis* 1994; 19: 867-83.

Patrick DL, Cheadle A, Thompson DC, Diehr P, Koepsell T, Kinne S. The validity of self-reported smoking: a review and meta analysis. *Am J Public Health* 1994; 84: 1086-93.

Péron Y, Strohmenger C. *Demographic and Health Indicators: Presentation and Interpretation.* Ottawa: Minister of Supply and Services Canada, 1985 (Catalogue No. 82-543E).

Petterson B, Nelson KB, Watson L, Stanley F. Twins, triplets, and cerebral palsy in births in Western Australia in the 1980's. *Br Med J* 1993; 307: 1239-43.

Postl B. Native health: it's time for action. *Can Med Assoc J* 1997; 157: 165-6.

Premature mortality due to congenital anomalies — United States. *MMWR* 1988; 37: 505-6.

Prysak M, Lorenz RP, Kisly A. Pregnancy outcome in nulliparous women 35 years and older. *Obstet Gynecol* 1995; 85: 65-70.

Renfrew MJ, Hannah W, Albers L, Floyd E. Practices that minimize trauma to the genital tract in childbirth: A systematic review of the literature. *Birth* 1998; 25: 143-60.

Reproductive Care Program of Nova Scotia. *Nova Scotia Atlee Perinatal Database Report: Maternal and Infant Discharges from January 1-December 31, 1997.* Halifax: 2000.

Rodis JF, Egan JF, Craffey A, Ciarleglio L, Greenstein RM, Scorza WE. Calculated risk of chromosomal abnormalities in twin gestations. *Obstet Gynecol* 1990; 76: 1037-41.

Sauve RS, Robertson C, Etches P, Byrne PJ, Dayer-Zamora V. Before viability: a geographically based outcome study of infants weighing 500 grams or less at birth. *Pediatrics* 1998; 101: 438-45.

Sepkowitz S. International rankings of infant mortality and the United States vital statistics natality data collecting system — failure and success. *Int J Epidemiol* 1995; 24: 583-8.

SIDS Fact Sheet. Assembly of First Nations. National Indian Brotherhood, 2000. (Available: www.afn.ca/Programs/Health%20Secretariat/sids_fact_sheet.htm).

Smith ME, Newcombe HB. Use of the Canadian Mortality Data Base for epidemiologic follow up. *Can J Public Health* 1982; 73: 39-45.

Society of Obstetricians and Gynaecologists of Canada. *Dystocia. Society of Obstetricians and Gynaecologists of Canada Policy Statement.* Ottawa: SOGC, 1995.

Society of Obstetricians and Gynaecologists of Canada. *Fetal Health Surveillance in Labour, Parts 1 through 4. Society of Obstetricians and Gynaecologists of Canada Policy Statement.* Ottawa: SOGC, 1995.

Society of Obstetricians and Gynaecologists of Canada. *Fetal Health Surveillance in Labour, Conclusion. Society of Obstetricians and Gynaecologists of Canada Policy Statement.* Ottawa: SOGC, 1996,

Society of Obstetricians and Gynaecologists of Canada. *Induction of Labour, SOGC Clinical Practice Guidelines for Obstetrics, Number 23.* Ottawa: SOGC, 1996.

Society of Obstetricians and Gynaecologists of Canada. *The Canadian Consensus Conference on Breech Management at Term. Society of Obstetricians and Gynaecologists of Canada Policy Statement.* Ottawa: SOGC, 1994.

Society of Obstetricians and Gynaecologists of Canada. *The SOGC consensus statement on the management of twin pregnancies. Part two: Report of focus group on impact of twin pregnancies.* Barrett J. (Ed.). (Available: www.sogc.org/multiple/sogcconsensus.htm)

Society of Obstetricians and Gynaecologists of Canada. *Vaginal Birth after a Previous Cesarean. Society of Obstetricians and Gynaecologists of Canada Policy Statement.* Ottawa: SOGC, 1993.

Statistics Canada. Births. *Vital Statistics* 1973; 1.

Statistics Canada. *Births and Deaths, 1991, 1992, 1993, 1994, 1995.* Ottawa: Statistics Canada, Health Statistics Division (Catalogue No. 84-210-XPB (annual)).

Statistics Canada. *Births and Deaths 1996, 1997.* Ottawa: Statistics Canada, Health Statistics Division, 1999 (Catalogue No. 84F0210-XPB (annual)).

Statistics Canada. Causes of Death, 1988. *Health Rep* 1990; (11S): 2(1).

Statistics Canada. Causes of Death, 1989. *Health Rep* 1991; (11S): 3(1).

Statistics Canada. *Causes of Death 1973, 1974, 1975, 1976, 1977, 1978, 1979, 1980, 1981, 1982, 1983, 1984, 1985, 1986, 1987.* Ottawa: Statistics Canada, Health Statistics Division (Catalogue No. 84-203-XPB (annual)).

Statistics Canada. *Causes of Death, 1990.* Ottawa: Statistics Canada, Health Statistics Division, 1992; (11S): 4(1).

Statistics Canada. *Causes of Death 1991, 1992, 1993, 1994, 1995, 1996, 1997.* Ottawa: Statistics Canada, Health Statistics Division (Catalogue No. 84-208-XPB (annual)).

Statistics Canada. *Statistical Report on the Health of Canadians.* Ottawa: Statistics Canada, 1999 (Catalogue No. 82-570-XPE).

Statistics Canada. *The Daily:* Friday, April 7, 2000.

Statistics Canada. *Therapeutic Abortions, 1995.* Ottawa: Statistics Canada, Health Statistics Division, 1997 (Catalogue No. 82-219-XPB).

Statistics Canada, Human Resources Development Canada. *National Longitudinal Survey of Children and Youth, Overview of the Survey Instruments for 1996-97 Data Collection, Cycle 2.* Ottawa: Statistics Canada, 1997 (Catalogue No. 89F0078-XPE).

Stoler JM, Huntington KS, Peterson CM, Peterson KP, Daniel P, Aboagye KK et al. The prenatal detection of significant alcohol exposure with maternal blood markers. *J Pediatr* 1998; 133: 346-52.

Sue-A-Quan AK, Hannah ME, Cohen MM, Foster GA, Liston RM. Effect of labour induction on rates of stillbirth and cesarean section in post-term pregnancies. *Can Med Assoc J* 1999; 160: 1145-9.

Svenson LW, Schopflocher DP, Sauve RS, Robertson CM. Alberta's infant mortality rate: the effect of the registration of live newborns weighing less than 500 g. *Can J Public Health* 1998; 89: 188-9.

Thomson M. Heavy birthweight in native Indians of British Columbia. *Can J Public Health* 1990; 81: 443-6.

Tuormaa TE. The adverse effects of tobacco smoking on reproduction and health: a review from the literature. *Nutr Health* 1995; 10: 105-20.

Turner LA, McCourt C. Folic acid fortification: what does it mean for patients and physicians? *Can Med Assoc J* 1998; 158: 773-6.

U.S. Department of Health and Human Services. *The Health Benefits of Smoking Cessation.* U.S. Department of Health and Human Services, Public Health Service, Centers for Disease Control, Center for Chronic Disease Prevention and Health Promotion, Office of Smoking and Health, 1990 (DHHS Publication No. (CDC) 90-8416).

Ventura SJ, Martin JA, Curtin SC, Mathews TJ. Births: Final Data for 1997. *National vital statistics reports;* vol 47 no. 18. Hyattsville, Maryland: National Center for Health Statistics, 1999.

Wen SW, Kramer MS, Liu S, Dzakpasu S, Sauve R for the Fetal and Infant Health Study Group. Infant mortality by gestational age and birth weight in Canadian provinces and territories, 1990-1994 births. *Chronic Dis Can* 2000; 21: 14-22.

Wen SW, Liu S, Fowler D. Trends and variations in neonatal length of in-hospital stay in Canada. *Can J Public Health* 1998; 89: 115-9.

Wen SW, Liu S, Joseph KS, Rouleau J, Allen A. Patterns of infant mortality caused by major congenital anomalies. *Teratology* 2000; 61: 342-6.

Wen SW, Liu S, Joseph KS, Trouton K, Allen A. Regional patterns of infant mortality caused by lethal congenital anomalies. *Can J Public Health* 1999; 90: 316-9.

Wen SW, Liu S, Marcoux S, Fowler D. Trends and variations in length of hospital stay for childbirth in Canada. *Can Med Assoc J* 1998; 158: 875-80.

Wen SW, Liu S, Marcoux S, Fowler D. Uses and limitations of routine hospital admission/ separation records for perinatal surveillance. *Chron Dis Can* 1997; 18: 113-9.

Werler MM. Teratogen update: smoking and reproductive outcomes. *Teratology* 1997; 55: 382-8.

Wilcox LS, Kiely JL, Melvin CL, Martin MC. Assisted reproductive technologies: estimates of their contribution to multiple births and newborn hospital days in the United States. *Fertil Steril* 1996; 65: 361-6.

Wilkins R. Mortality by neighbourhood income in urban Canada, 1986-1991. Presentation at the Canadian Society for Epidemiology and Biostatistics, Newfoundland, Canada, August 1995.

Wilkins R, Adams O, Branker A. Changes in mortality by income in urban Canada from 1971 to 1986. *Health Rep* 1989; 1: 137-74.

World Health Organization. *International Statistical Classification of Diseases and Related Health Problems*, 10th Revision. Vol. 2. Geneva: WHO, 1993: 129-33.

World Health Organization. *Manual of the International Statistical Classification of Diseases, Injuries, and Causes of Death*. Based on the Recommendation of the Ninth Revision Conference, 1975, Geneva.

World Health Organization. *Manual of the International Statistical Classification of Diseases, Injuries, and Causes of Death*, 9th Revision. Vol. 1. Geneva: WHO, 1977.

World Health Organization/UNICEF. *Revised 1990 Estimates of Maternal Mortality: A New Approach by WHO and UNICEF*. Geneva: WHO, 1991.

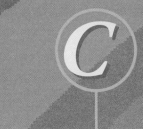

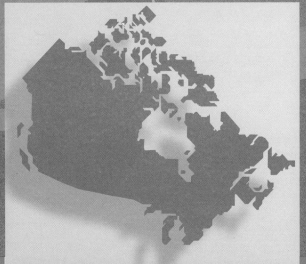

Appendices

Appendix A

Data Sources and Methods

Data Sources

The principal data sources for this perinatal health report were vital statistics, hospitalization data and the National Longitudinal Survey of Children and Youth (NLSCY). Population estimates and abortion statistics from Statistics Canada, as well as other peer-reviewed research were also used. Table A1 lists the principal data sources for each indicator presented in this report. Following the table is a description of each principal data source.

Table A1 **Principal data sources for each indicator**

Indicator	Data source		
	Vital statistics	Hospitalization	NLSCY
Prevalence of prenatal smoking			x
Prevalence of prenatal alcohol consumption			x
Prevalence of breastfeeding			x
Rate of live births to teenagers	x		
Rate of live births to older mothers	x		
Labour induction rate		x	
Cesarean section rate		x	
Rate of operative vaginal deliveries		x	
Rate of trauma to the perineum		x	
Rate of early maternal discharge from hospital after childbirth		x	
Rate of early neonatal discharge from hospital after birth		x	
Maternal mortality ratio	x		
Induced abortion ratio*	x	x	
Ectopic pregnancy rate		x	
Severe maternal morbidity ratio		x	
Rate of maternal readmission after discharge following childbirth		x	
Preterm birth rate	x		
Postterm birth rate	x		
Fetal growth: small-for-gestational-age rate, large-for-gestational-age rate	x		
Fetal and infant mortality rates	x		
Severe neonatal morbidity rate		x	
Multiple birth rate	x	x	
Prevalence of congenital anomalies	x	x	
Rate of neonatal hospital readmission after discharge at birth		x	

* Includes abortions performed in abortion clinics.

87

Vital Statistics

Registration of births and deaths is compulsory under provincial and territorial *Vital Statistics Acts* or equivalent legislation. While the provincial and territorial *Vital Statistics Acts* may vary slightly among the provinces and territories, they follow a model *Vital Statistics Act* that was developed to promote uniformity of legislation and reporting among the provinces and territories. Every year, the provinces and territories send their birth, stillbirth and death registration data to Statistics Canada. Statistics Canada compiles these data into national databases of births, stillbirths and deaths, called the Canadian Vital Statistics System.[1-4]

The Canadian Vital Statistics System covers all births and deaths occurring in Canada. Births and deaths of Canadian residents occurring in the United States are also included, being reported under a reciprocal agreement. However, births and deaths of Canadian residents occurring in countries other than Canada and the United States are not reported.[1] The preparation and maintenance of these national databases requires incorporation of late registrations and amendments, as well as the elimination of duplicate registrations.

As part of the Canadian Perinatal Surveillance System (CPSS) initiative, Statistics Canada, under contract to the Bureau of Reproductive and Child Health, has developed a mechanism by which information on live births and infant deaths will be linked from 1985 onwards.[5] With the permission of the provinces and territories, the resulting birth-infant death linked analysis file is an important data source for CPSS analyses. This file has personal identifiers removed.

The birth and death statistics in this report may differ slightly from those previously published by Statistics Canada, as a result of updates to the data files.

Data Quality

There are numerous strengths of national vital statistics data. Coverage for births and deaths in the Canadian Vital Statistics System is nearly complete. Due to the large number of records, analysis within subpopulations is possible. An additional strength is that the legislation for the collection of vital statistics data is similar across all provinces and territories, as are data forms, definitions and collection methods. Data are also available at the individual level and can therefore be linked to other data sources. Finally, causes of death are coded to an international classification.[6]

A major limitation of national vital statistics data is that data are not available on as timely a basis as would be desirable. Currently, the last year of available data is 1997, which became available to the CPSS in the second half of 1999. Additional limitations relate to the quality or completeness of some variables. For example, due to concerns about the quality of gestational age and birth weight data in Ontario, Ontario data were excluded from indicators which use these variables. There may also be a small undercount in the number of live births reported for Ontario each year. Data for Newfoundland in the national birth database were incomplete prior to 1991; consequently, Newfoundland data were excluded from temporal trends. Finally, cause of death information may not always incorporate the results of coroner and medical examiner investigations.

Hospitalization Data

Three sources of hospitalization data were utilized: the Canadian Institute for Health Information's (CIHI's) Discharge Abstract Database (DAD), Manitoba Health's Perinatal Surveillance Database and the Canadian Congenital Anomalies Surveillance System (CCASS).

Canadian Institute for Health Information's Discharge Abstract Database

CIHI maintains the DAD which captures hospital separation — transfer, discharge or death — from the majority of Canada's acute care hospitals. The DAD is an electronic database that includes information on inpatient acute, chronic and rehabilitation care and day surgery, accounting for about 85% of all acute care inpatient discharges in Canada. The information is obtained directly from participating hospitals.[7] The DAD contains considerable data on each hospitalization, including demographic and residence information, length of stay, most responsible diagnosis, secondary and co-morbid diagnoses and procedures performed during the hospitalization. Diagnoses are coded in the DAD according to the International Classification of Diseases, Ninth Revision (ICD-9) and procedures coded according to the Canadian Classification of Diagnostic, Therapeutic and Surgical Procedures (CCP). The DAD also categorizes hospitalizations by case mix group (CMG), a classification according to diagnosis and intensity of care required.

Internal record linkage of the obstetric delivery record, the newborn record and the readmission record in the DAD was performed to provide information on neonatal and maternal readmission.

Data Quality

The Bureau of Reproductive and Child Health investigated and evaluated the DAD to see if it could serve the needs of a national perinatal surveillance system.[8,9] The quality of data for delivering mothers and their newborns recorded in the DAD from April 1, 1984 to March 31, 1995 was examined. The number of illogical and out-of-range values in the CIHI data was found to be low, the occurrence of maternal and infant diseases estimated from the data was similar to that in the literature, and major medical or obstetric complications recorded in the DAD were good predictors of adverse pregnancy outcomes.[8]

Major diagnoses and procedures appear to be well captured; however, complex or obscure diagnoses are likely coded variably. Accuracy is also likely to be lower for codes other than the primary or most responsible diagnosis. CIHI is undertaking a quality assurance study of the DAD that will involve comparison of information in charts with information coded in the DAD for a sample of hospitals. The CPSS is collaborating with CIHI to expand this study to include specific maternal and newborn diagnoses.

In addition to the general limitation of potential coding errors, there are several other problems in using the DAD for national perinatal surveillance:

- Out-of-hospital births are not captured.

- Pregnancies with non-birth outcomes (e.g., terminations) may not be captured.

- The DAD does not include all hospital admissions/separations in Canada. Québec data are not included in the DAD, and data for Manitoba and Nova Scotia are not complete for some years. Indicators which were calculated using hospitalization data therefore exclude Nova Scotia and Manitoba from temporal trends. Québec data are excluded from both interprovincial/territorial comparisons and temporal trends using hospitalization data.

- Currently, the DAD does not capture information on gestational age and parity.

Manitoba Health's Perinatal Surveillance Database

Statistics based on hospitalization data from Manitoba were calculated by Manitoba Health, using its Perinatal Surveillance Database. The following description of the database was obtained from Manitoba Health.

The bulk of the data was obtained by linking obstetrical hospital records and newborn hospital records dated April 1, 1984 to March 31, 1997. The Manitoba Health hospital records were searched for obstetrical (mother) or newborn admissions. The obstetrical and newborn records were linked together by hospital of admission, mother's hospital record number, newborn's hospital record number, Manitoba Health family registration number and surname. Extensive verification of the linkage was conducted in the cases where mother's surname was not the same as the newborn's surname. Most data lines contain both mother and newborn information. Those mother records that did not link to a newborn record were retained only if one of the mother's diagnoses included a stillborn v-code (V271, V274, V277), assuming that a newborn record was not created for these births. All newborn records were retained because a newborn record represented a birth regardless of whether a link could be made with a maternal record. Manitoba Health medical coverage data were merged with the linked records by a newborn's personal health identification number (PHIN) to add cancel codes and dates to this database.

The linked obstetrical-newborn database only identifies pregnancies that resulted in a live birth or a stillbirth. To capture pregnancies which did not result in a birth, the Manitoba Health hospital records were again searched, and all obstetrical admissions regardless of outcome were summarized into a pregnancy database. Using this pregnancy database it was possible to calculate rates of reported ectopic pregnancies, molar pregnancies, spontaneous abortions (miscarriages) and induced abortions, in addition to stillbirths and live births.

Data Quality

Manitoba Health hospital records share many of the features and limitations of the data in the DAD. For example, pregnancies resulting in a home birth, an induced abortion at a private clinic, or an unreported spontaneous abortion are not captured in this database.

Canadian Congenital Anomalies Surveillance System

CCASS data are largely culled from the DAD. Additional data sources are also relied upon, particularly to provide coverage of provinces poorly represented by the DAD. The Manitoba hospitalization database is used in Manitoba, and Québec data are from the Système de maintenance et d'exploitation des données pour l'étude de la clientèle hospitalière (Med-Écho); these two systems are similar to the DAD. Alberta uses its own reporting system, the Alberta Congenital Anomalies Surveillance System (ACASS). The primary sources of data for ACASS are vital statistics, hospital reporting and special communications with genetics clinics, specialty paediatric clinics and laboratories.

Data Quality

The definition, interpretation and diagnosis of an anomaly can differ from one physician to another. Certain anomalies can be excluded or included, and others are not always evaluated against the same criteria, which can make reporting varied and inaccurate. Some anomalies may be reported as part of a syndrome or may be reported separately. All of these circumstances can produce variations in rates nationally, provincially or even locally. Other factors contributing to inaccuracies are trends and variations in use of prenatal diagnosis and pregnancy termination and in hospitalization practices. Prenatally diagnosed fetuses with congenital anomalies that are aborted are not included in the CCASS because the DAD does not capture them. Hospitalization practices directly influence the potential of discovering new cases of congenital anomalies with the DAD data.

The data provided by Alberta, Manitoba and Québec are not from the same source and, therefore, are subject to their own limitations, including the ones mentioned in the paragraph above. Another limitation of CCASS DAD-based data is the possibility of duplicate data, since records of separate admissions of the same infant with sometimes different congenital anomalies are present in the DAD. Despite the fact that the records for the same infant are linked together, this process is successful only if the relevant variables, such as date of birth, sex, scrambled health insurance number, postal or geographic code and ICD-9 codes, are present and accurate. The accuracy and completeness of these variables can vary and create inflated rates for some areas.

Other limitations of the DAD data are that they only cover births that occur in hospitals and not all hospitals participate in the DAD. Additional limitations include the lack of exposure and behaviour risk factors and mother's past and current pregnancy history; these data are nonexistent in the CCASS. Other factors, such as coding, transcription and classification errors, can also contribute to discrepancies in rates of congenital anomalies.

National Longitudinal Survey of Children and Youth[10]

The primary objective of the NLSCY is to develop a national database on the characteristics and life experiences of Canadian children as they grow from infancy to adulthood. The survey is conducted by Statistics Canada and collects cross-sectional information as well as longitudinal data. Data collection began in 1994-1995 and will be repeated every two years to follow the children surveyed in 1994-1995. In subsequent years, a cross-sectional sample will be added for age groups no longer covered by the longitudinal sample.

The public use microdata file of the 1996-1997 data collection cycle was used for analyses. This file does not include data from the territories. Information on prenatal smoking and alcohol consumption, and breastfeeding was available for 7,040 children 0-3 years old, representing approximately 284,000 children when weighted. All rates were calculated using sample weights.

Data Quality

The survey is primarily designed for national-, regional- and some provincial/territorial-level analysis. Analysis of subpopulations is limited by insufficient sample sizes. Attrition may further reduce the sample size in subsequent data collection cycles. Perinatal health information was often not detailed enough to be used for in-depth analysis, and it may be subject to incorrect recall because it was collected retrospectively up to three years after the birth of the child. Perinatal health information may also be subject to a small selection bias because it was collected only for children still living at the time the sample was selected.

Methods

Statistical methods were primarily descriptive, including frequencies, rates, percentages and means. Where events were rare or rates were based on a small sample, caution should be exercised in interpreting results. Records with key information missing were excluded from analyses. In the birth-infant death linked file, all live births at < 22 weeks and < 500 g were assumed to have died on the first day of life and were classified as such.

Statistics presented for most indicators consist of:

1. **Temporal trends at the national level** — The time period covered in the temporal trends dates back as far as 1981, depending on the data sources used and the particular indicator. If complete provincial data were not available for all years of a temporal trend, data from that province were excluded from the Canadian rates. In some cases, where events were rare, data for several years were aggregated.

2. **Interprovincial/territorial comparisons** — Interprovincial/territorial comparisons are presented for the most recent year for which data were available. In some cases, regional differences are assessed and interpreted using standard errors and 95% confidence intervals. Separate statistics could not be calculated for Nunavut as the time period covered in this report preceded the creation of this new territory.

3. **Comparisons by maternal age** — Some indicators are analyzed by maternal age, where available and appropriate.

The majority of indicators are presented graphically. However, data tables corresponding to all figures are presented in Appendix E.

References

1. Statistics Canada. *Births and Deaths 1996, 1997*. Ottawa: Statistics Canada, Health Statistics Division, 1999 (Catalogue No. 84F0210-XPB (annual)).

2. Fair M. The development of national vital statistics in Canada: Part 1 — From 1605 to 1945. *Health Rep* 1994; 6: 355-68.

3. Fair M, Cyr M. The Canadian Birth Data Base: a new research tool to study reproductive outcomes. *Health Rep* 1993; 5: 281-90.

4. Smith ME, Newcombe HB. Use of the Canadian Mortality Data Base for epidemiologic follow up. *Can J Public Health* 1982; 73: 39-45.

5. Fair M, Cyr M, Allen AC, Wen SW, Guyon G, MacDonald RC et al. *Validation Study for a Record Linkage of Births and Infant Deaths in Canada*. Ottawa: Statistics Canada, 1999 (Catalogue No. 84F0013-XIE).

6. World Health Organization. *Manual of the International Statistical Classification of Diseases, Injuries and Causes of Death.* Based on the Recommendation of the Ninth Revision Conference, 1975, Geneva.

7. Canadian Institute for Health Information. Website (www.cihi.ca). Accessed February 7, 2000.

8. Wen SW, Liu S, Marcoux S, Fowler D. Uses and limitations of routine hospital admission/separation records for perinatal surveillance. *Chron Dis Can* 1997; 18: 113-9.

9. Liu S, Wen SW. Development of record linkage of hospital discharge data for the study of neonatal readmission. *Chron Dis Can* 1999; 20: 77-81.

10. Statistics Canada, Human Resources Development Canada. *National Longitudinal Survey of Children and Youth, Overview of the Survey Instruments for 1996-97 Data Collection, Cycle 2.* Ottawa: Statistics Canada, 1997 (Catalogue No. 89F0078-XPE).

Appendix B

List of Perinatal Health Indicators

Additional Perinatal Health Indicators

Appendix C

List of Acronyms

ACASS	Alberta Congenital Anomalies Surveillance System
ARBD	alcohol-related birth defect
CCASS	Canadian Congenital Anomalies Surveillance System
CCP	Canadian Classification of Diagnostic, Therapeutic and Surgical Procedures
CI	confidence interval
CIHI	Canadian Institute for Health Information
CMG	case mix group
CPS	Canadian Paediatric Society
CPSS	Canadian Perinatal Surveillance System
CS	cesarean section
DAD	Discharge Abstract Database
DC	Dieticians of Canada
FAS	fetal alcohol syndrome
ICD-9	International Classification of Diseases, Ninth Revision
IUGR	intrauterine growth restriction
LGA	large for gestational age
Med-Écho	Système de maintenance et d'exploitation des données pour l'étude de la clientèle hospitalière
MMR	maternal mortality ratio
NLSCY	National Longitudinal Survey of Children and Youth
NTD	neural tube defect
PHIN	personal health identification number
RDS	respiratory distress syndrome
SD	standard deviation
SGA	small for gestational age
SOGC	Society of Obstetricians and Gynaecologists of Canada
UNICEF	United Nations Children's Fund
VBAC	vaginal birth after cesarean
WHO	World Health Organization

Appendix D

Components of Fetal-Infant Mortality*

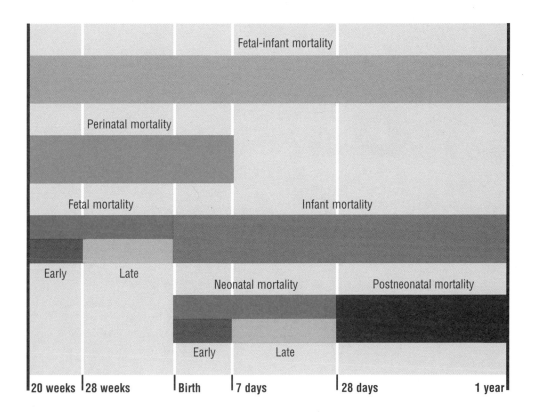

* Adapted from Péron Y, Strohmenger C. *Demographic and Health Indicators: Presentation and Interpretation.*
Ottawa: Minister of Supply and Services Canada, 1985 (Catalogue No. 82-543E); and Monnier A. Les méthodes
d'analyse de la mortalité infantile. In: *Manuel d'analyse de la mortalité.* Paris: INED, 1985: 52-5.

In calculating the fetal-infant mortality rate, perinatal mortality rate and stillbirth rate, the denominator reflects total
births (live births and stillbirths), whereas in calculating the infant mortality rate, neonatal mortality rate (early and
late) and postneonatal mortality rate, the denominator includes only live births.

Appendix E

List of Data Tables

Data Tables

Table E1.1 **Prevalence of selected maternal behaviours, by maternal age and region/province,** *Canada (excluding the territories),[†] 1996-1997*

Percent of children aged 0-3 years whose mother reported selected behaviours

	Prenatal smoking	Prenatal alcohol consumption	Breastfeeding Any breast-feeding	Breastfed at least three months*
Maternal age (years)				
< 20	40.5**	—	72.5	31.6**
20-24	33.5	11.7***	70.7	38.9
25-29	24.5	14.1	74.1	47.7
30-34	16.9	16.4	79.4	59.1
≥ 35	17.2	22.6	78.2	59.2
Region/Province				
Atlantic Provinces	25.2	7.7**	65.3	40.6
Québec	25.8	24.9	57.7	34.8
Ontario	18.8	13.8	81.2	59.2
Prairie Provinces	21.0	16.1	88.0	63.2
British Columbia	18.6	14.9	89.0	65.2
CANADA[†]	**21.3**	**16.6**	**76.7**	**53.6**

Source: Statistics Canada. National Longitudinal Survey of Children and Youth (Public Use Microdata Files), 1996-1997.

† Data for the territories are not available in the Public Use Microdata Files. Percentages were calculated from a sample of 7,040 children weighted to represent approximately 284,000 children 0-3 years old.

* Children less than three months old were excluded from "breastfed at least three months" calculations.

** Estimate is based on a small sample size.

*** Further categorization of age was not possible due to a small sample size. Estimate based on population < 25.

Table E1.2 **Number of live births, by maternal age,**

Canada (excluding Newfoundland), 1981-1997*

Year	10-14 years	15-19 years	20-24 years	25-29 years	30-34 years	35-39 years	40-44 years	45-49 years	50-54 years	Number of births unknown age	Total live births
1981	268	29,054	110,535	135,581	67,668	15,328	2,080	113	3	457	361,087
1982	281	28,258	109,915	136,880	68,704	17,092	2,113	95	2	216	363,556
1983	222	25,377	107,199	139,651	71,506	18,293	2,111	100	0	181	364,640
1984	248	23,635	103,226	143,031	75,847	19,977	2,181	85	1	151	368,382
1985	225	22,089	98,257	143,817	79,109	21,040	2,317	82	1	165	367,102
1986	210	21,448	92,905	143,545	81,422	22,414	2,536	85	0	144	364,709
1987	235	20,975	86,576	142,700	84,567	23,695	2,863	100	2	164	361,877
1988	224	21,075	83,415	146,013	89,269	25,847	3,283	106	1	14	369,247
1989	214	22,479	83,070	150,727	96,513	28,134	3,567	96	1	22	384,823
1990	239	23,175	81,727	154,257	103,352	31,064	3,856	99	0	42	397,811
1991	261	23,370	78,735	147,530	106,132	32,720	4,072	135	0	2,407	395,362
1992	255	23,215	75,827	143,042	109,853	34,589	4,495	106	3	333	391,718
1993	249	22,783	73,458	133,163	110,735	36,349	4,809	139	5	274	381,964
1994	239	23,117	71,654	127,493	112,222	38,134	5,232	129	13	534	378,767
1995	232	22,863	69,634	119,968	113,122	40,060	5,593	192	2	483	372,149
1996	221	21,065	66,149	114,784	109,554	42,249	6,014	204	4	206	360,450
1997	214	19,208	62,291	108,379	103,729	42,679	6,334	207	3	127	343,171

Source: Statistics Canada. Canadian Vital Statistics System, 1981-1997.

* Newfoundland is excluded because data are not available nationally prior to 1991.

Table E1.3 **Number of females, by age,**

Canada (excluding Newfoundland), 1981-1997*

Year	10-14 years	15-19 years	20-24 years	25-29 years	30-34 years	35-39 years	40-44 years	45-49 years	50-54 years
1981	912,514	1,126,623	1,200,228	1,096,612	1,011,583	801,399	658,347	611,182	612,637
1982	900,493	1,087,206	1,206,223	1,132,310	1,018,188	859,743	680,386	611,049	615,857
1983	890,157	1,036,757	1,208,099	1,158,596	1,032,397	903,098	710,081	613,125	616,357
1984	879,227	988,796	1,206,945	1,174,705	1,056,864	940,317	739,933	622,900	614,207
1985	870,361	952,515	1,196,540	1,185,387	1,088,432	975,230	769,788	633,454	610,541
1986	859,698	938,235	1,169,683	1,200,402	1,117,845	1,004,374	804,885	649,427	609,125
1987	862,801	925,569	1,127,939	1,216,479	1,151,278	1,018,661	862,386	675,066	607,687
1988	868,625	920,019	1,078,365	1,232,886	1,179,953	1,044,862	907,981	709,155	609,612
1989	880,788	918,194	1,046,999	1,254,392	1,211,740	1,083,214	955,249	743,764	621,877
1990	890,472	916,469	1,018,392	1,249,956	1,236,814	1,121,282	1,000,838	776,940	635,391
1991	901,471	910,497	1,001,166	1,212,408	1,258,909	1,149,248	1,039,446	813,224	655,438
1992	915,144	911,820	992,553	1,176,907	1,268,587	1,182,540	1,049,562	871,527	680,688
1993	929,615	915,955	981,417	1,131,569	1,279,302	1,213,249	1,070,253	920,355	713,443
1994	942,994	927,831	973,231	1,091,747	1,284,201	1,237,836	1,100,021	966,378	746,575
1995	951,014	940,270	967,452	1,062,096	1,278,105	1,260,509	1,134,954	1,010,283	779,258
1996	957,088	955,491	965,195	1,048,730	1,252,834	1,284,677	1,167,632	1,046,014	814,456
1997	962,692	965,064	970,964	1,040,734	1,222,368	1,301,633	1,206,279	1,057,933	873,955

Source: Statistics Canada. Canadian female population estimates, 1981-1997.

* Newfoundland is excluded because data are not available nationally prior to 1991.

Table E1.4 | **Percent of live births, by maternal age,**
Canada (excluding Newfoundland),* 1981-1997

Year	10-14 years	15-19 years	20-24 years	25-29 years	30-34 years	35-39 years	40-44 years	45-54 years
1981	0.07	8.06	30.65	37.60	18.76	4.25	0.58	0.03
1982	0.08	7.78	30.25	37.67	18.91	4.70	0.58	0.03
1983	0.06	6.96	29.41	38.32	19.62	5.02	0.58	0.03
1984	0.07	6.42	28.03	38.84	20.60	5.43	0.59	0.02
1985	0.06	6.02	26.78	39.19	21.56	5.73	0.63	0.02
1986	0.06	5.88	25.48	39.37	22.33	6.15	0.70	0.02
1987	0.06	5.80	23.93	39.45	23.38	6.55	0.79	0.03
1988	0.06	5.71	22.59	39.54	24.18	7.00	0.89	0.03
1989	0.06	5.84	21.59	39.17	25.08	7.31	0.93	0.03
1990	0.06	5.83	20.55	38.78	25.98	7.81	0.97	0.02
1991	0.07	5.95	20.04	37.54	27.01	8.33	1.04	0.03
1992	0.07	5.93	19.37	36.55	28.07	8.84	1.15	0.03
1993	0.07	5.97	19.25	34.89	29.01	9.52	1.26	0.04
1994	0.06	6.11	18.94	33.71	29.67	10.08	1.38	0.04
1995	0.06	6.15	18.74	32.28	30.44	10.78	1.50	0.05
1996	0.06	5.85	18.36	31.86	30.41	11.73	1.67	0.06
1997	0.06	5.60	18.16	31.59	30.24	12.44	1.85	0.06

Source: Statistics Canada. Canadian Vital Statistics System, 1981-1997.

* Newfoundland is excluded because data are not available nationally prior to 1991.

Table E1.5 | **Age-specific live birth rates per 1,000 females,**
Canada (excluding Newfoundland),* 1981-1997

Year	10-14 years	15-19 years	20-24 years	25-29 years	30-34 years	35-39 years	40-44 years	45-49 years	50-54 years
1981	0.29	25.79	92.10	123.64	66.89	19.13	3.16	0.18	0.00
1982	0.31	25.99	91.12	120.89	67.48	19.88	3.11	0.16	0.00
1983	0.25	24.48	88.73	120.53	69.26	20.26	2.97	0.16	0.00
1984	0.28	23.90	85.53	121.76	71.77	21.24	2.95	0.14	0.00
1985	0.26	23.19	82.12	121.32	72.68	21.57	3.01	0.13	0.00
1986	0.24	22.86	79.43	119.58	72.84	22.32	3.15	0.13	0.00
1987	0.27	22.66	76.76	117.31	73.45	23.26	3.32	0.15	0.00
1988	0.26	22.91	77.35	118.43	75.65	24.74	3.62	0.15	0.00
1989	0.24	24.48	79.34	120.16	79.65	25.97	3.73	0.13	0.00
1990	0.27	25.29	80.25	123.41	83.56	27.70	3.85	0.13	0.00
1991	0.29	25.67	78.64	121.68	84.30	28.47	3.92	0.17	0.00
1992	0.28	25.46	76.40	121.54	86.59	29.25	4.28	0.12	0.00
1993	0.27	24.87	74.85	117.68	86.56	29.96	4.49	0.15	0.01
1994	0.25	24.92	73.62	116.78	87.39	30.81	4.76	0.13	0.02
1995	0.24	24.32	71.98	112.95	88.51	31.78	4.93	0.19	0.00
1996	0.23	22.05	68.53	109.45	87.44	32.89	5.15	0.20	0.00
1997	0.22	19.90	64.15	104.14	84.86	32.79	5.25	0.20	0.00

Sources: Statistics Canada. Canadian Vital Statistics System, 1981-1997.
Statistics Canada. Canadian female population estimates, 1981-1997.

* Newfoundland is excluded because data are not available nationally prior to 1991.

Table E2.1 **Number and rate of labour inductions, by province/territory,**
Canada (excluding Québec), 1997-1998*

Province/Territory	Number of labour inductions	Number of hospital deliveries	Inductions (95% CI) per 100 hospital deliveries	
Newfoundland	1,047	5,290	19.8	(18.7-20.9)
Prince Edward Island	277	1,481	18.7	(16.7-20.7)
Nova Scotia	1,974	9,756	20.2	(19.4-21.0)
New Brunswick	1,295	7,963	16.3	(15.5-17.1)
Ontario	24,170	135,616	17.8	(17.6-18.0)
Manitoba	2,918	14,833	19.7	(19.0-20.3)
Saskatchewan	2,703	12,318	21.9	(21.2-22.7)
Alberta	8,024	36,254	22.1	(21.7-22.6)
British Columbia	7,171	43,529	16.5	(16.1-16.8)
Yukon	64	427	15.0	(11.7-18.7)
Northwest Territories	122	1,166	10.4	(8.7-12.3)
CANADA*	**49,765**	**268,633**	**18.5**	**(18.4-18.7)**

Sources: Canadian Institute for Health Information. Discharge Abstract Database, 1997-1998.
Manitoba Health, Epidemiology Unit. Perinatal Surveillance Database, 1997-1998.
* Québec data are not included in the Discharge Abstract Database (DAD).
CI — confidence interval.

Table E2.2 **Number and rate of total and primary cesarean sections (CS),**
Canada (excluding Québec, Nova Scotia and Manitoba), 1994-1995 to 1997-1998*

Year	Number of CS	Number of hospital deliveries	CS per 100 hospital deliveries	Number of primary CS	Number of births, no previous CS	Primary CS per 100 hospital deliveries
1994-1995	47,394	266,055	17.8	30,463	241,372	12.6
1995-1996	47,194	261,834	18.0	30,312	236,438	12.8
1996-1997	46,682	250,593	18.6	30,187	225,796	13.4
1997-1998	46,513	244,044	19.1	30,241	219,676	13.8

Source: Canadian Institute for Health Information. Discharge Abstract Database, 1994-1995 to 1997-1998.
* Québec data are not included in the DAD. Nova Scotia and Manitoba are excluded because complete data for all years are not available in the DAD.

Table E2.3 **Number and rate of repeat cesarean sections (CS),**
Canada (excluding Québec, Nova Scotia and Manitoba), 1994-1995 to 1997-1998*

Year	Number of women with previous CS	Number of hospital deliveries	Percent of women with a previous CS	Number of repeat CS	Percent of CS among women with a previous CS
1994-1995	24,683	266,055	9.3	16,931	68.6
1995-1996	25,396	261,834	9.7	16,882	66.5
1996-1997	24,797	250,593	9.9	16,495	66.5
1997-1998	24,368	244,044	10.0	16,272	66.8

Source: Canadian Institute for Health Information. Discharge Abstract Database, 1994-1995 to 1997-1998.
* Québec data are not included in the DAD. Nova Scotia and Manitoba are excluded because complete data for all years are not available in the DAD.
** The observed increase over time in the percent of women with previous cesarean delivery may be due to an increased tendency to record previous cesarean delivery in the hospital discharge abstract.

Table E2.4 **Number and rate of operative vaginal deliveries, by province/territory,** *Canada (excluding Québec),* 1997-1998*

Province/Territory	Number of operative vaginal deliveries	Number of hospital vaginal deliveries	Operative vaginal deliveries (95% CI) per 100 hospital vaginal deliveries	
Newfoundland	730	4,051	18.0	(16.8-19.2)
Prince Edward Island	115	1,170	9.8	(8.2-11.7)
Nova Scotia	1,074	7,936	13.5	(12.8-14.3)
New Brunswick	1,130	6,207	18.2	(17.2-19.2)
Ontario	20,780	109,856	18.9	(18.7-19.1)
Manitoba	979	12,392	7.9	(7.4-8.4)
Saskatchewan	1,925	10,360	18.5	(17.8-19.3)
Alberta	5,642	30,272	18.6	(18.2-19.0)
British Columbia	5,125	34,221	14.9	(14.6-15.3)
Yukon	56	364	15.4	(11.8-19.5)
Northwest Territories	55	1,030	5.3	(4.0-6.9)
CANADA*	**37,611**	**217,859**	**17.2**	**(17.1-17.4)**

Sources: Canadian Institute for Health Information. Discharge Abstract Database, 1997-1998.
　　　　Manitoba Health, Epidemiology Unit. Perinatal Surveillance Database, 1997-1998.

* Québec data are not included in the DAD.

CI — confidence interval.

Table E2.5 **Number and rate of vaginal deliveries by forceps, by province/territory,** *Canada (excluding Québec),* 1997-1998*

Province/Territory	Number of forceps deliveries	Number of hospital vaginal deliveries	Forceps use (95% CI) per 100 hospital vaginal deliveries	
Newfoundland	350	4,051	8.6	(7.8-9.5)
Prince Edward Island	53	1,170	4.5	(3.4-5.9)
Nova Scotia	677	7,936	8.5	(7.9-9.1)
New Brunswick	550	6,207	8.8	(8.2-9.6)
Ontario	8,925	109,856	8.1	(8.0-8.3)
Manitoba	358	12,392	2.9	(2.6-3.2)
Saskatchewan	541	10,360	5.2	(4.8-5.6)
Alberta	2,250	30,272	7.4	(7.1-7.7)
British Columbia	2,325	34,221	6.8	(6.5-7.1)
Yukon	4	364	1.1	(0.3-2.8)
Northwest Territories	12	1,030	1.2	(0.6-2.0)
CANADA*	**16,045**	**217,859**	**7.4**	**(7.2-7.5)**

Sources: Canadian Institute for Health Information. Discharge Abstract Database, 1997-1998.
　　　　Manitoba Health, Epidemiology Unit. Perinatal Surveillance Database, 1997-1998.

* Québec data are not included in the DAD.

CI — confidence interval.

Table E2.6 **Number and rate of vaginal deliveries by vacuum extractions, by province/territory,** *Canada (excluding Québec),* 1997-1998

Province/Territory	Number of vacuum extractions	Number of hospital vaginal deliveries	Vacuum extractions (95% CI) per 100 hospital vaginal deliveries	
Newfoundland	387	4,051	9.5	(8.7-10.5)
Prince Edward Island	67	1,170	5.7	(4.5-7.2)
Nova Scotia	407	7,936	5.1	(4.7-5.6)
New Brunswick	698	6,207	11.2	(10.5-12.0)
Ontario	12,411	109,856	11.3	(11.1-11.5)
Manitoba	621	12,392	5.0	(4.6-5.4)
Saskatchewan	1,534	10,360	14.8	(14.1-15.5)
Alberta	3,778	30,272	12.5	(12.1-12.8)
British Columbia	2,972	34,221	8.7	(8.4-9.0)
Yukon	53	364	14.6	(11.1-18.6)
Northwest Territories	43	1,030	4.2	(3.0-5.6)
CANADA*	**22,971**	**217,859**	**10.5**	**(10.4-10.7)**

Sources: Canadian Institute for Health Information. Discharge Abstract Database, 1997-1998.
Manitoba Health, Epidemiology Unit. Perinatal Surveillance Database, 1997-1998.

* Québec data are not included in the DAD.

CI — confidence interval.

Table E2.7 **Number and rate of perineal lacerations,**
Canada (excluding Québec, Nova Scotia and Manitoba), 1989-1990 to 1997-1998

Year	Number of first- and second-degree lacerations	Number of third- and fourth-degree lacerations	Number of hospital vaginal deliveries	First- and second-degree lacerations per 100 hospital vaginal deliveries	Third- and fourth-degree lacerations per 100 hospital vaginal deliveries
1989-1990	63,784	8,188	213,440	29.9	3.8
1990-1991	70,453	9,085	221,711	31.8	4.1
1991-1992	77,950	9,175	223,236	34.9	4.1
1992-1993	86,255	8,962	220,579	39.1	4.1
1993-1994	92,228	8,611	217,595	42.4	4.0
1994-1995	97,735	8,599	218,661	44.7	3.9
1995-1996	100,092	7,934	214,640	46.6	3.7
1996-1997	98,190	7,875	203,911	48.2	3.9
1997-1998	96,477	7,527	197,531	48.8	3.8

Source: Canadian Institute for Health Information. Discharge Abstract Database, 1989-1990 to 1997-1998.

* Québec data are not included in the Discharge Abstract Database. Nova Scotia and Manitoba are excluded because complete data for all years are not available in the DAD.

Table E2.8 **Number and rate of episiotomies,**

Canada, 1989-1990 to 1997-1998*

Year	Number of episiotomies	Number of hospital vaginal deliveries	Episiotomies per 100 hospital vaginal deliveries
1989-1990	173,128	314,936	55.0
1990-1991	169,077	328,364	51.5
1991-1992	157,093	328,601	47.8
1992-1993	139,259	327,250	42.6
1993-1994	121,405	321,857	37.7
1994-1995	No data**	218,661	No data**
1995-1996	No data**	214,640	No data**
1996-1997	55,118	203,911	27.0
1997-1998	50,140	197,531	25.4

Sources: Canadian Institute for Health Information. Discharge Abstract Database, 1989-1997.
　　　　Graham et al., 1997.

* 1996-1997 to 1997-1998 episiotomy data exclude Québec, Nova Scotia and Manitoba. Québec data
　are not included in the DAD. Nova Scotia and Manitoba are excluded because complete data for all years
　are not available in the DAD.

** There are no available episiotomy data for 1994-1995 or 1995-1996.

Table E2.9 **Number and rate of episiotomies, by province/territory,**

Canada (excluding Québec), 1997-1998*

Province/Territory	Number of episiotomies	Number of hospital vaginal deliveries	Episiotomies (95% CI) per 100 hospital vaginal deliveries	
Newfoundland	1,091	4,051	26.9	(25.6-28.3)
Prince Edward Island	411	1,170	35.1	(32.4-37.9)
Nova Scotia	2,073	7,936	26.1	(25.2-27.1)
New Brunswick	1,994	6,207	32.1	(31.0-33.3)
Ontario	30,479	109,856	27.7	(27.5-28.0)
Manitoba	2,678	12,392	21.6	(20.9-22.3)
Saskatchewan	2,383	10,360	23.0	(22.2-23.8)
Alberta	6,680	30,272	22.1	(21.6-22.5)
British Columbia	7,004	34,221	20.5	(20.0-20.9)
Yukon	22	364	6.0	(3.8-9.0)
Northwest Territories	76	1,030	7.4	(5.9-9.1)
CANADA*	**54,891**	**217,859**	**25.2**	**(25.0-25.4)**

Sources: Canadian Institute for Health Information. Discharge Abstract Database, 1997-1998.
　　　　Manitoba Health, Epidemiology Unit. Perinatal Surveillance Database, 1997-1998.

* Québec data are not included in the DAD.

CI — confidence interval.

Table E2.10 **Number and rate of short maternal length of stay (LOS) for childbirth (vaginal and cesarean deliveries),** *Canada (excluding Québec, Nova Scotia and Manitoba),* 1989-1990 to 1997-1998*

Year	Vaginal deliveries LOS < 2 days			Cesarean deliveries LOS < 4 days		
	Number of women with LOS < 2 days	Number of hospital deliveries	Hospital deliveries with LOS < 2 days per 100 hospital vaginal deliveries	Number of women with LOS < 4 days	Number of hospital deliveries	Hospital deliveries with LOS < 4 days per 100 hospital cesarean deliveries
1989-1990	6,801	213,440	3.2	1,099	52,336	2.1
1990-1991	7,781	221,711	3.5	1,337	53,073	2.5
1991-1992	10,071	223,236	4.5	1,685	51,347	3.3
1992-1993	13,276	220,579	6.0	2,736	49,741	5.5
1993-1994	1,954	217,595	9.0	4,647	48,456	9.6
1994-1995	36,294	218,661	16.6	8,174	47,394	17.3
1995-1996	47,593	214,640	22.2	10,962	47,194	23.2
1996-1997	46,788	203,911	23.0	12,295	46,682	26.3
1997-1998	50,495	197,531	25.6	14,556	46,513	31.3

Source: Canadian Institute for Health Information. Discharge Abstract Database, 1989-1990 to 1997-1998.

* Québec data are not included in the DAD. Nova Scotia and Manitoba are excluded because complete data for all years are not available in the DAD.

Table E2.11 **Number and rate of short maternal length of stay (LOS) for childbirth (vaginal deliveries), by province/territory,** *Canada (excluding Québec),* 1997-1998*

Province/Territory	Number of women with LOS < 2 days	Number of hospital vaginal deliveries	Hospital deliveries (95% CI) with LOS < 2 days per 100 hospital vaginal deliveries	
Newfoundland	215	4,051	5.3	(4.6-6.0)
Prince Edward Island	18	1,170	1.5	(0.9-2.4)
Nova Scotia	1,097	7,936	13.8	(13.1-14.6)
New Brunswick	240	6,207	3.9	(3.4-4.4)
Ontario	31,247	109,856	28.4	(28.2-28.7)
Manitoba**	1,113	11,712	9.5	(9.0-10.1)
Saskatchewan	974	10,360	9.4	(8.8-10.0)
Alberta	10,988	30,272	36.3	(35.8-36.8)
British Columbia	6,540	34,221	19.1	(18.7-19.5)
Yukon	44	364	12.1	(8.9-15.9)
Northwest Territories	229	1,030	22.2	(19.7-24.9)
CANADA*	**52,705**	**217,179**	**24.3**	**(24.1-24.4)**

Sources: Canadian Institute for Health Information. Discharge Abstract Database, 1997-1998.
 Manitoba Health, Epidemiology Unit. Perinatal Surveillance Database, 1997-1998.

* Québec data are not included in the DAD.

** Manitoba LOS data are missing for some hospital deliveries; therefore, the number of deliveries included in these analyses differs from that in Table E2.9.

CI — confidence interval.

Table E2.12 **Number and rate of short maternal length of stay (LOS) for childbirth (cesarean deliveries), by province/territory,** *Canada (excluding Québec)*, 1997-1998*

Province/Territory	Cesarean delivery LOS < 4 days		
	Number of women with LOS < 4 days	Number of hospital cesarean deliveries	Hospital deliveries (95% CI) with LOS < 4 days per 100 cesarean deliveries
Newfoundland	196	1,239	15.8 (13.8-18.0)
Prince Edward Island	14	311	4.5 (2.5-7.4)
Nova Scotia	607	1,820	33.4 (31.2-35.6)
New Brunswick	461	1,756	26.3 (24.2-28.4)
Ontario	7,877	25,760	30.6 (30.0-31.1)
Manitoba	513	2,433	21.1 (19.5-22.8)
Saskatchewan	421	1,958	21.5 (19.7-23.4)
Alberta	2,692	5,982	45.0 (43.7-46.3)
British Columbia	2,849	9,308	30.6 (29.7-31.6)
Yukon	20	63	31.7 (20.6-44.7)
Northwest Territories	26	136	19.1 (12.9-26.7)
CANADA*	**15,676**	**50,766**	**30.9 (30.5-31.3)**

Sources: Canadian Institute for Health Information. Discharge Abstract Database, 1997-1998.
      Manitoba Health, Epidemiology Unit. Perinatal Surveillance Database, 1997-1998.

* Québec data are not included in the DAD.

CI — confidence interval.

Table E2.13 **Number and rate of early neonatal discharge from hospital after birth,** *Canada (excluding Québec, Nova Scotia and Manitoba),* 1989-1990 to 1997-1998*

Year	Birth weight 1,000-2,499 g			Birth weight ≥ 2,500 g		
	Number of newborns with LOS < 2 days	Number of hospital live births	Newborns with LOS < 2 days per 100 hospital live births	Number of newborns with LOS < 2 days	Number of hospital live births	Newborns with LOS < 2 days per 100 hospital live births
1989-1990	1,519	13,566	11.2	7,942	252,782	3.1
1990-1991	1,419	13,824	10.3	9,864	261,811	3.8
1991-1992	1,454	13,989	10.4	13,255	261,480	5.1
1992-1993	1,504	13,774	10.9	18,399	257,731	7.1
1993-1994	1,600	13,820	11.6	27,187	253,274	10.7
1994-1995	1,975	14,235	13.9	49,353	253,065	19.5
1995-1996	2,078	13,866	15.0	62,804	249,093	25.2
1996-1997	1,885	13,252	14.2	61,741	238,656	25.9
1997-1998	1,771	12,974	13.7	66,735	232,509	28.7

Source: Canadian Institute for Health Information. Discharge Abstract Database, 1989-1990 to 1997-1998.

* Québec data are not included in the DAD. Nova Scotia and Manitoba are excluded because complete data for all years are not available in the DAD.

LOS — length of stay.

Table E2.14 **Number and rate of early neonatal discharge from hospital after birth, by province/territory,** *Canada (excluding Québec),* 1997-1998*

Province/Territory	Birth weight 1,000-2,499 g			Birth weight ≥ 2,500 g		
	Number of newborns LOS with < 2 days	Number of hospital live births	Newborns (95% CI) with LOS < 2 days per 100 hospital live births	Number of newborns with LOS < 2 days	Number of hospital live births	Newborns (95% CI) with LOS < 2 days per 100 hospital live births
Newfoundland	39	288	13.5 (9.8-18.0)	364	5,020	7.3 (6.5-8.0)
Prince Edward Island	7	59	11.9 (4.9-22.9)	21	1,432	1.5 (0.9-2.2)
Nova Scotia	33	545	6.1 (4.2-8.4)	1,655	9,310	17.8 (17.0-18.6)
New Brunswick	12	396	3.0 (1.6-5.2)	294	7,627	3.9 (3.4-4.3)
Ontario	914	7,356	12.4 (11.7-13.2)	40,159	129,102	31.1 (30.9-31.4)
Manitoba	37	698	5.3 (3.8-7.2)	1,771	13,216	13.4 (12.8-14.0)
Saskatchewan	43	589	7.3 (5.3-9.7)	1,441	11,837	12.2 (11.6-12.8)
Alberta	330	2,131	15.5 (14.0-17.1)	14,803	34,362	43.1 (42.6-43.6)
British Columbia	416	2,103	19.8 (18.1-21.5)	9,273	41,584	22.3 (21.9-22.7)
Yukon	1	14	7.1 (0.2-33.9)	55	417	13.2 (10.1-16.8)
Northwest Territories	9	38	23.7 (11.4-40.2)	325	1,128	28.8 (26.2-31.6)
CANADA*	**1,841**	**14,217**	**12.9 (12.4-13.5)**	**70,161**	**255,035**	**27.5 (27.3-27.7)**

Sources: Canadian Institute for Health Information. Discharge Abstract Database, 1997-1998.
　　　　Manitoba Health, Epidemiology Unit. Perinatal Surveillance Database, 1997-1998.

* Québec data are not included in the DAD.

CI — confidence interval.

Table E3.1 **Number of maternal deaths and maternal mortality ratios (MMR), by direct and indirect causes,** *Canada, for five-year intervals, 1973-1977 to 1993-1997*

	Number of maternal deaths				Maternal deaths per 100,000 live births	
Five-year interval	Due to direct causes	Due to indirect causes	Total	Number of live births in interval	Due to direct causes only	Due to direct and indirect causes
1973-1977	141	N/A*	141	1,715,649	8.2	8.2
1978-1982	98	10	108	1,790,281	5.5	6.0
1983-1987	69	4	73	1,827,244	3.8	4.0
1988-1992	71	4	75	1,953,259	3.6	3.8
1993-1997	75	8	83	1,866,315	3.4	4.4

Sources: see chapter 3, p. 41, references 3-10.

*A definition of indirect obstetric death first appeared in the Ninth Revision of the International Classification of Diseases system and deaths classified as indirect maternal deaths were first included in cause of death tabulations in Canada in 1980.

Table E3.2 | **Number, ratio and rate of induced abortions,**

Canada, 1990-1997

Year	Number of induced abortions*	Number of live births	Number of females 15-44 years	Induced abortions (95% CI) per 100 live births		Induced abortions (95% CI) per 1,000 females 15-44 years	
1990	92,901	405,486	6,543,751	22.9	(22.8-23.0)	14.0	(14.1-14.3)
1991	95,059	402,528	6,717,442	23.6	(23.5-23.7)	14.2	(14.1-14.2)
1992	102,085	398,636	6,727,276	25.6	(25.5-25.7)	15.2	(15.1-15.3)
1993	104,403	388,386	6,736,358	26.9	(26.7-27.0)	15.5	(15.4-15.6)
1994	106,255	385,108	6,756,678	27.6	(27.4-27.7)	15.7	(15.6-15.8)
1995	108,248	378,008	6,782,196	28.2	(28.5-28.8)	16.0	(15.9-16.1)
1996	111,659	366,198	6,809,887	30.5	(30.3-30.6)	16.4	(16.3-16.5)
1997	114,848	348,587	6,838,788	32.9	(32.8-33.1)	16.8	(16.7-16.9)

Sources: Statistics Canada, *Therapeutic Abortions, 1995.*
Statistics Canada. Canadian Vital Statistics System, 1990-1997.
Statistics Canada. *The Daily:* Friday, April 7, 2000.
Statistics Canada. Canadian female population estimates, 1990-1997.

* Includes induced abortions to women under 15 and over 44 years of age performed in hospitals and clinics and in the U.S.A.

CI — confidence interval.

Table E3.3 | **Number, ratio and rate of induced abortions, by province/territory,**

Canada,* 1997

Province/Territory	Number of induced abortions*	Number of live births	Number of females 15-44 years	Induced abortions (95% CI) per 100 live births		Induced abortions (95% CI) per 1,000 females 15-44 years	
Newfoundland	838	5,416	132,252	15.5	(14.5-16.5)	6.3	(5.9-6.8)
Prince Edward Island	151	1,591	30,165	9.5	(8.1-11.0)	5.0	(4.2-5.9)
Nova Scotia	2,045	9,952	212,088	20.5	(19.8-21.4)	9.6	(9.2-10.1)
New Brunswick	1,113	7,922	171,780	14.0	(13.3-14.8)	6.5	(6.1-6.9)
Québec	28,186	79,772	1,648,490	35.3	(35.0-35.7)	17.1	(16.9-17.3)
Ontario	47,174	132,997	2,574,867	35.5	(35.2-35.7)	18.3	(18.2-18.5)
Manitoba	3,626	14,655	247,916	24.7	(24.0-25.4)	14.6	(14.2-15.1)
Saskatchewan	1,996	12,859	219,790	15.5	(14.9-16.2)	9.1	(8.7-9.5)
Alberta	10,337	36,905	672,011	28.0	(27.6-28.5)	15.4	(15.1-15.7)
British Columbia	15,583	44,576	904,811	35.0	(34.5-35.4)	17.2	(17.0-17.5)
Yukon	121	474	8,130	25.5	(21.7-29.7)	14.9	(12.4-17.8)
Northwest Territories	317	1,468	16,488	21.6	(19.5-23.8)	19.2	(17.2-21.4)
CANADA*	**114,848**	**348,587**	**6,838,788**	**32.9**	**(32.8-33.1)**	**16.8**	**(16.7-16.9)**

Sources: Statistics Canada. *The Daily:* Friday, April 7, 2000.
Statistics Canada. Canadian Vital Statistics System, 1997.
Statistics Canada. *Births and Deaths, 1997 (shelf tables).*

* Includes induced abortions to women under 15 and over 44 years of age performed in hospitals and clinics and in the U.S.A.

CI — confidence interval.

Table E3.4 **Number and rate of age-specific induced abortions,**

Canada, 1997

Age	Number of induced abortions	Number of females†	Induced abortions (95% CI) per 1,000 females	
Unknown age	3,547	—	—	—
< 15**	519	196,530	2.6	(2.4-2.9)
15-19	21,204	987,083	21.5	(21.2-21.8)
20-24	33,640	992,280	33.9	(33.5-34.3)
25-29	23,963	1,061,261	22.6	(22.3-22.9)
30-34	17,422	1,243,426	14.0	(13.8-14.2)
35-39	10,975	1,323,672	8.3	(8.1-8.4)
40-44***	3,578	1,228,711	2.9	(2.8-3.0)
All ages*	**114,848**	**6,836,433**	**16.8**	**(16.7-16.9)**

Sources: Canadian Institute for Health Information. Therapeutic Abortion Survey, 1997.
Statistics Canada. Health Statistics Division, March 2000.

* Includes abortions performed in hospitals, clinics and in the U.S.A. Also includes abortions to women over 44 years. Totals include cases with age not specified. Totals include 293 abortions to Canadian women in the U.S.A.

** Rates based on women aged 14 years.

*** Includes induced abortions to women over 44 years of age at pregnancy termination. Rates based on female population aged 40-44 years.

† Population data vary from other tables because they are taken from Canadian Institute for Health Information, Therapeutic Abortion Survey, 1997.

CI — confidence interval.

Table E3.5 **Number and rate of ectopic pregnancies,**

Canada (excluding Québec, Nova Scotia and Manitoba), 1989-1990 to 1997-1998

Year	Number of ectopic pregnancies	Number of reported pregnancies**	Ectopic pregnancies per 1,000 reported pregnancies
1989-1990	5,732	295,563	19.4
1990-1991	6,003	302,983	19.8
1991-1992	5,866	301,110	19.5
1992-1993	5,913	294,412	20.1
1993-1994	5,536	286,651	19.3
1994-1995	5,336	284,792	18.7
1995-1996	5,057	278,231	18.2
1996-1997	4,717	265,358	17.8
1997-1998	4,315	257,480	16.8

Source: Canadian Institute for Health Information. Discharge Abstract Database, 1989-1990 to 1997-1998

* Québec data are not included in the DAD. Nova Scotia and Manitoba are excluded because complete data for all years are not available in the DAD.

** Reported pregnancies include live births, stillbirths, hospital-based induced abortions and ectopic pregnancies.

Table E3.6 | **Number and rate of ectopic pregnancies, by province/territory,**
Canada (excluding Québec),* 1997-1998

Province/Territory	Number of ectopic pregnancies	Number of reported pregnancies**	Ectopic pregnancies (95% CI) per 1,000 reported pregnancies	
Newfoundland	96	5,706	16.8	(13.6-20.5)
Prince Edward Island	19	1,546	12.3	(7.4-19.1)
Nova Scotia	123	10,090	12.2	(10.1-14.5)
New Brunswick	123	8,414	14.6	(12.2-17.4)
Ontario	2,213	141,614	15.6	(15.0-16.3)
Manitoba	342	20,576	16.6	(14.9-18.5)
Saskatchewan	217	13,112	16.5	(14.4-18.9)
Alberta	746	39,187	19.0	(17.7-20.4)
British Columbia	849	46,149	18.4	(17.2-19.7)
Yukon	18	474	38.0	(22.7-59.4)
Northwest Territories	34	1,278	26.6	(18.5-37.0)
CANADA*	**4,780**	**288,146**	**16.6**	**(16.1-17.1)**

Sources: Canadian Institute for Health Information. Discharge Abstract Database, 1997-1998.
Manitoba Health, Epidemiology Unit. Perinatal Surveillance Database, 1997-1998.

* Québec data are not included in the DAD.

** Reported pregnancies include live births, stillbirths, hospital-based induced abortions and ectopic pregnancies to all women.

CI — confidence interval.

Table E3.7 | **Number and rate of ectopic pregnancies, by maternal age,**
Canada (excluding Québec),* 1997-1998

Age	Number of ectopic pregnancies	Number of reported pregnancies**	Ectopic pregnancies (95% CI) per 1,000 reported pregnancies	
15-19	234	18,775	12.5	(10.9-14.2)
20-24	716	52,932	13.5	(12.6-14.5)
25-29	1,287	88,126	14.6	(13.8-15.4)
30-34	1,474	85,238	17.3	(16.4-18.2)
35-39	862	36,864	23.4	(21.9-25.0)
40-44	195	5,934	32.9	(28.5-37.7)
45-49	12	216	55.6	(29.0-95.0)
Total (15-49)	**4,780**	**288,085**	**16.6**	**(16.1-17.1)**

Sources: Canadian Institute for Health Information. Discharge Abstract Database, 1997-1998.
Manitoba Health, Epidemiology Unit. Perinatal Surveillance Database, 1997-1998.

* Québec data are not included in the DAD.

** Reported pregnancies include live births, stillbirths, hospital-based induced abortions and ectopic pregnancies to women 15-49 years old only.

CI — confidence interval.

Table E3.8 **Number and rate of maternal readmissions within three months of discharge from hospital following childbirth,*** *Canada (excluding Québec, Nova Scotia and Manitoba),*** 1990-1991 to 1997-1998*

Year	Vaginal deliveries			Cesarean deliveries		
	Number of readmissions	Number of hospital deliveries	Readmissions per 100 hospital deliveries	Number of readmissions	Number of hospital deliveries	Readmissions per 100 hospital deliveries
1990-1991	5,055	199,710	2.5	1,526	48,367	3.2
1991-1992	5,068	201,839	2.5	1,581	46,870	3.4
1992-1993	5,595	206,752	2.7	1,607	46,781	3.4
1993-1994	5,490	206,248	2.7	1,691	46,157	3.7
1994-1995	5,578	207,678	2.7	1,752	45,271	3.9
1995-1996	5,219	203,084	2.6	1,758	44,394	4.0
1996-1997	4,880	194,288	2.5	1,664	44,514	3.7
1997-1998	4,672	191,390	2.4	1,747	44,888	3.9

Source: Canadian Institute for Health Information. Discharge Abstract Database, 1990-1991 to 1997-1998.

* Women who were directly transferred after childbirth and women with initial LOS > 20 days were excluded from analysis.

**Québec data are not included in the DAD. Nova Scotia and Manitoba are excluded because complete data for all years are not available in the DAD.

Table E3.9 **Number and rate of maternal readmissions within three months of discharge from hospital following childbirth (vaginal deliveries),*** **by province/territory,** *Canada (excluding Québec),*** 1995-1996 to 1997-1998*

Province/Territory	Number of readmissions	Number of hospital deliveries	Readmissions (95% CI) per 100 hospital deliveries	
Newfoundland	470	12,677	3.7	(3.4-4.1)
Prince Edward Island	73	3,728	2.0	(1.5-2.5)
Nova Scotia	590	22,348	2.7	(2.4-2.9)
New Brunswick	575	18,855	3.1	(2.8-3.3)
Ontario	6,782	333,454	2.0	(2.0-2.1)
Manitoba	1,386	40,946	2.6	(3.2-3.6)
Saskatchewan	530	21,944	2.5	(2.2-2.6)
Alberta	3,373	90,673	3.7	(3.6-3.8)
British Columbia	2,777	104,349	2.7	(2.6-2.8)
Northwest Territories	127	3,251	4.0	(3.3-4.6)
CANADA*	**16,683**	**652,225**	**2.6**	**(2.5-2.6)**

Sources: Canadian Institute for Health Information. Discharge Abstract Database, 1995-1996 to 1997-1998.
  Manitoba Health, Epidemiology Unit. Perinatal Surveillance Database, 1995-1996 to 1997-1998.

* Women who were directly transferred after childbirth and women with initial LOS > 20 days were excluded from analysis.

** Québec data are not included in the DAD.

CI — confidence interval.

Table E3.10 **Number and rate of maternal readmissions within three months of discharge from hospital following childbirth (cesarean deliveries),* by province/territory,** *Canada (excluding Québec),** 1995-1996 to 1997-1998*

Province/Territory	Number of readmissions	Number of hospital deliveries	Readmissions (95% CI) per 100 hospital deliveries	
Newfoundland	174	3,533	4.9	(4.2-5.7)
Prince Edward Island	42	996	4.2	(3.1-5.7)
Nova Scotia	260	5,244	5.0	(4.4-5.6)
New Brunswick	267	5,019	5.3	(4.7-6.0)
Ontario	2,418	74,630	3.3	(3.1-3.4)
Manitoba	306	7,990	3.8	(3.4-4.3)
Saskatchewan	160	4,302	3.9	(3.2-4.3)
Alberta	942	17,229	5.5	(5.1-5.8)
British Columbia	1,081	27,721	4.0	(3.7-4.1)
Northwest Territories	19	381	4.9	(3.0-7.7)
CANADA*	**5,669**	**147,045**	**3.9**	**(3.8-4.0)**

Sources: Canadian Institute for Health Information. Discharge Abstract Database, 1995-1996 to 1997-1998.
   Manitoba Health, Epidemiology Unit. Perinatal Surveillance Database, 1995-1996 to 1997-1998.

* Women who were directly transferred to other institutions after childbirth and women with initial LOS > 20 days were excluded from analysis.

** Québec data are not included in the DAD.

CI — confidence interval.

Table E3.11 **Number of maternal readmissions within three months of discharge from hospital following childbirth,* by primary diagnosis,** *Canada (excluding Québec),** 1995-1996 to 1997-1998*

Primary diagnosis at readmission (ICD-9 code)	Mode of delivery (number)		
	All	Cesarean	Vaginal
1. Postpartum hemorrhage (666)	3,229	383	2,846
2. Cholelithiasis (574)	2,948	646	2,302
3. Major puerperal infection (670)	2,258	578	1,680
4. Other and unspecified complications of the puerperium, not elsewhere classified (674)	1,601	1,159	442
5. Postpartum care and examination (V24)	812	247	565
6. Persons seeking consultation without complaint of sickness (V65)	786	85	701
7. Infection of the breast and nipple associated with childbirth (675)	692	108	584
8. Other current conditions in the mother classifiable elsewhere, but complicating pregnancy, childbirth, or the puerperium(648)	498	130	368
9. Complications of pregnancy, not elsewhere classified (646)	522	137	385
10. Symptoms involving abdomen and pelvis (789)	419	101	318
11. Encounter for contraceptive management (V25)	337	21	316
12. Complications of procedures, not elsewhere classified (998)	267	137	130
13. Venous complications in pregnancy and the puerperium (671)	250	89	161
14. Other diagnoses	7,733	1,848	5,885
Total	**22,352**	**5,669**	**16,683**

Source: Canadian Institute for Health Information. Discharge Abstract Database, 1995-1996 to 1997-1998.
   Manitoba Health, Epidemiology Unit. Perinatal Surveillance Database, 1995-1996 to 1997-1998.

* Women who were directly transferred after childbirth and women with initial LOS > 20 days were excluded from analysis.

** Québec data are not included in the DAD.

Table E4.1 **Number and rate of preterm births,**
Canada (excluding Ontario and Newfoundland), 1981-1997*

Year	Number of preterm births	Number of live births**	Preterm births per 100 live births
1981	15,292	238,059	6.4
1982	14,961	238,231	6.3
1983	14,689	237,686	6.2
1984	15,146	236,929	6.4
1985	14,199	234,869	6.1
1986	14,097	229,773	6.1
1987	14,310	227,102	6.3
1988	15,342	229,925	6.7
1989	15,321	235,475	6.5
1990	16,129	244,215	6.6
1991	15,956	240,421	6.6
1992	15,877	238,077	6.7
1993	15,262	231,988	6.6
1994	15,655	231,295	6.8
1995	15,707	225,578	7.0
1996	15,439	218,775	7.1
1997	14,773	208,999	7.1

Source: Statistics Canada. Canadian Vital Statistics System, 1981-1997.

* Ontario is excluded due to data quality concerns. Newfoundland is excluded because data are not available nationally prior to 1991.

** Excludes live births with unknown gestational age and gestational age < 20 weeks.

Table E4.2 **Number and rate of preterm births (singleton and multiple births),** *Canada (excluding Ontario),* 1997*

Birth order	Number of preterm births	Number of live births**	Preterm births per 100 live births
Singleton births	12,391	209,243	5.9
Twin births	2,556	4,953	51.6
Triplet or higher-order births	209	218	95.9
All live births	15,156	214,414	7.1

Source: Statistics Canada. Canadian Vital Statistics System, 1997.

* Ontario is excluded due to data quality concerns.

** Excludes live births with unknown gestational age and gestational age < 20 weeks.

Table E4.3 **Number and rate of preterm births, by province/territory,**
Canada (excluding Ontario), 1997*

Province/Territory	Number of preterm births	Number of live births**	Preterm births (95% CI) per 100 live births	
Newfoundland	401	5,415	7.4	(6.7-8.1)
Prince Edward Island	96	1,591	6.0	(4.9-7.3)
Nova Scotia	728	9,950	7.3	(6.8-7.8)
New Brunswick	490	7,922	6.2	(5.7-6.7)
Québec	5,750	78,728	7.3	(7.1-7.5)
Manitoba	1,084	14,648	7.4	(7.0-7.8)
Saskatchewan	872	12,859	6.8	(6.4-7.2)
Alberta	2,663	36,905	7.2	(7.0-7.5)
British Columbia	2,924	44,460	6.6	(6.3-6.8)
Yukon	29	474	6.1	(4.1-8.7)
Northwest Territories	119	1,462	8.1	(6.8-9.7)
CANADA*	**15,156**	**214,414**	**7.1**	**(7.0-7.2)**

Source: Statistics Canada. Canadian Vital Statistics System, 1997.

* Ontario is excluded due to data quality concerns.

** Excludes live births with unknown gestational age and gestational age < 20 weeks.

CI — confidence interval.

Table E4.4 **Number and rate of postterm births,**
Canada (excluding Ontario and Newfoundland), 1988-1997*

Year	Number of postterm births	Number of total births**	Postterm births per 100 total births
1988	10,033	231,231	4.3
1989	11,283	236,901	4.8
1990	11,268	245,596	4.6
1991	10,542	241,838	4.4
1992	8,931	239,451	3.7
1993	8,957	233,234	3.8
1994	7,237	232,560	3.1
1995	5,646	226,874	2.5
1996	4,305	219,946	2.0
1997	3,883	210,196	1.8

Source: Statistics Canada. Canadian Vital Statistics System, 1988-1997.

* Ontario is excluded due to data quality concerns. Newfoundland is excluded because data are not available nationally prior to 1991.

** Excludes live births and stillbirths with unknown gestational age and gestational age < 20 weeks.

Table E4.5 **Number and rate of postterm births, by province/territory,** *Canada (excluding Ontario),* 1997*

Province/Territory	Number of postterm births	Total births**	Postterm births (95% CI) per 100 total births	
Newfoundland	49	5,446	0.9	(0.7-1.2)
Prince Edward Island	50	1,596	3.1	(2.3-4.1)
Nova Scotia	473	10,018	4.7	(4.3-5.2)
New Brunswick	206	7,969	2.6	(2.2-3.0)
Québec	701	79,056	0.9	(0.8-1.0)
Manitoba	456	14,746	3.1	(2.8-3.4)
Saskatchewan	335	12,919	2.6	(2.3-2.9)
Alberta	726	37,151	2.0	(1.8-2.1)
British Columbia	892	44,785	2.0	(1.9-2.1)
Yukon	24	481	5.0	(3.2-7.3)
Northwest Territories	20	1,475	1.4	(0.8-2.1)
CANADA*	**3,932**	**215,642**	**1.8**	**(1.8-1.9)**

Source: Statistics Canada. Canadian Vital Statistics System, 1997.

* Ontario is excluded due to data quality concerns.

** Excludes live births and stillbirths with unknown gestational age and gestational age < 20 weeks.

CI — confidence interval.

Table E4.6 **Numbers and rates of small-for-gestational-age (SGA) and large-for-gestational-age (LGA) babies,** *Canada (excluding Ontario and Newfoundland),* 1988-1997*

Year	Number of SGA babies	Number of LGA babies	Number of live births**	SGA babies per 100 live births	LGA babies per 100 live births
1988	23,123	22,364	228,797	10.1	9.8
1989	23,698	22,448	234,549	10.1	9.6
1990	23,855	24,015	243,303	9.8	9.9
1991	23,047	23,961	239,414	9.6	10.0
1992	21,192	25,324	237,223	8.9	10.7
1993	21,436	23,919	231,229	9.3	10.3
1994	21,022	23,984	231,104	9.1	10.4
1995	20,419	23,292	224,195	9.1	10.4
1996	18,653	24,273	217,681	8.6	11.2
1997	17,895	22,230	207,758	8.6	10.7

Source: Statistics Canada. Canadian Vital Statistics System, 1988-1997.

* Ontario is excluded due to data quality concerns. Newfoundland is excluded because data are not available nationally prior to 1991.

** Excludes live births with unknown gestational age and birthweight, and gestational age < 20 weeks.

Table E4.7 **Numbers and rates of small-for-gestational-age (SGA) and large-for-gestational-age (LGA) babies, by province/territory,** *Canada (excluding Ontario),* 1997*

Province/Territory	Number of SGA babies	Number of LGA babies	Number of live births**	SGA babies (95% CI) per 100 live births		LGA babies (95% CI) per 100 live births	
Newfoundland	425	763	5,406	7.9	(7.2-8.6)	14.1	(13.2-15.1)
Prince Edward Island	125	238	1,585	7.9	(6.6-9.3)	15.0	(13.3-16.9)
Nova Scotia	866	1,274	9,942	8.7	(8.2-9.3)	12.8	(12.2-13.5)
New Brunswick	673	1,019	7,921	8.5	(7.9-9.1)	12.9	(12.1-13.6)
Québec	6,853	7,292	77,520	8.8	(8.6-9.0)	9.4	(9.2-9.6)
Manitoba	1,202	1,940	14,646	8.2	(7.8-8.7)	13.2	(12.7-13.8)
Saskatchewan	1,014	1,522	12,858	7.9	(7.4-8.4)	11.8	(11.3-12.4)
Alberta	3,429	3,751	36,901	9.3	(9.0-9.6)	10.2	(9.9-10.5)
British Columbia	3,595	4,949	44,453	8.1	(7.8-8.3)	11.1	(10.8-11.4)
Yukon	47	56	474	9.9	(7.4-13.0)	11.8	(9.0-15.1)
Northwest Territories	91	189	1,458	6.2	(5.1-7.6)	13.0	(11.3-14.8)
CANADA*	**18,320**	**22,993**	**213,164**	**8.6**	**(8.5-8.7)**	**10.8**	**(10.7-10.9)**

Source: Statistics Canada. Canadian Vital Statistics System, 1997.

* Ontario is excluded due to data quality concerns.

** Excludes live births with unknown gestational age and birthweight, and gestational age < 20 weeks.

CI — confidence interval.

Table E4.8 **Number and rate* of fetal deaths,**
*Canada (excluding Ontario and Newfoundland),** 1988-1997*

Year	Number of fetal deaths	Total births	Deaths per 1,000 total births
1988	1,128	232,321	4.86
1989	1,252	240,778	5.20
1990	1,213	248,117	4.89
1991	1,189	245,073	4.85
1992	1,152	242,277	4.75
1993	1,112	235,233	4.73
1994	1,122	232,825	4.82
1995	1,080	226,968	4.76
1996	981	221,422	4.43
1997	1,008	211,182	4.77

Source: Statistics Canada. Canadian Vital Statistics System, 1988-1997.

*Fetal death rates were based on all births excluding those with known birth weight of < 500 grams.

** Ontario is excluded due to data quality concerns. Newfoundland is excluded because data are not available nationally prior to 1991.

Table E4.9 **Number and rate* of fetal deaths, by province/territory,**
Canada (excluding Ontario),** 1997

Province/Territory	Number of fetal deaths	Total births	Fetal deaths (95% CI) per 1,000 total births	
Newfoundland	29	5,445	5.3	(3.6-7.6)
Prince Edward Island	4	1,595	2.5	(0.7-6.4)
Nova Scotia	56	10,008	5.6	(4.2-7.3)
New Brunswick	34	7,956	4.3	(3.0-6.0)
Québec	340	80,112	4.2	(3.8-4.7)
Manitoba	62	14,717	4.2	(3.2-5.4)
Saskatchewan	58	12,917	4.5	(3.4-5.8)
Alberta	179	37,084	4.8	(4.1-5.6)
British Columbia	257	44,833	5.7	(5.1-6.5)
Yukon	6	480	12.5	(4.6-27.0)
Northwest Territories	12	1,480	8.1	(4.2-14.1)
CANADA	**1,037**	**216,627**	**4.8**	**(4.5-5.1)**

Source: Statistics Canada. Canadian Vital Statistics System, 1997.
*Fetal death rates were based on all births excluding those with known birth weight of < 500 grams.
** Ontario is excluded due to data quality concerns.
CI — confidence interval.

Table E4.10 **Number and rate of neonatal (0-27 days) deaths,**
Canada (excluding Newfoundland),* 1988-1997

Year	Number of neonatal deaths	Number of live births	Deaths per 1,000 live births
1988	1,718	369,247	4.65
1989	1,827	384,823	4.75
1990	1,822	397,811	4.58
1991	1,605	395,362	4.06
1992	1,540	391,718	3.93
1993	1,577	381,964	4.13
1994	1,598	378,767	4.22
1995	1,550	372,149	4.16
1996	1,409	360,450	3.91
1997	1,336	343,171	3.89

Source: Statistics Canada. Canadian Vital Statistics System, 1988-1997.
* Newfoundland is excluded because data are not available nationally prior to 1991.

Table E4.11 **Number and rate of neonatal (0-27 days) deaths, by province/territory,** *Canada, 1997*

Province/Territory	Number of neonatal deaths	Number of live births	Deaths (95% CI) per 1,000 live births	
Newfoundland	22	5,416	4.1	(2.5-6.1)
Prince Edward Island	4	1,591	2.5	(0.7-6.4)
Nova Scotia	34	9,952	3.4	(2.4-4.8)
New Brunswick	30	7,922	3.8	(2.6-5.4)
Québec	311	79,772	3.9	(3.5-4.4)
Ontario	518	132,997	3.9	(3.6-4.2)
Manitoba	71	14,655	4.8	(3.8-6.1)
Saskatchewan	77	12,859	6.0	(4.7-7.5)
Alberta	128	36,905	3.5	(2.9-4.1)
British Columbia	151	44,576	3.4	(2.9-4.0)
Yukon	2	474	4.2	(0.5-15.2)
Northwest Territories	10	1,468	6.8	(3.3-12.5)
CANADA	**1,358**	**348,587**	**3.9**	**(3.7-4.1)**

Source: Statistics Canada. Canadian Vital Statistics System, 1997.
CI — confidence interval.

Table E4.12 **Number and rate of postneonatal (28-364 days) deaths,** *Canada (excluding Newfoundland),* 1988-1997*

Year	Number of postneonatal deaths	Number of infants ≥ 28 days old	Deaths per 1,000 infants ≥ 28 days old
1988	985	367,529	2.68
1989	967	382,996	2.52
1990	874	395,989	2.21
1991	912	393,757	2.32
1992	841	390,178	2.16
1993	819	380,388	2.15
1994	768	377,171	2.04
1995	725	370,599	1.96
1996	604	359,042	1.68
1997	563	341,835	1.65

Source: Statistics Canada. Canadian Vital Statistics System, 1988-1997.

* Newfoundland is excluded because data are not available nationally prior to 1991.

Table E4.13 **Number and rate of postneonatal (28-364 days) deaths, by province/territory,** *Canada, 1997*

Province/Territory	Number of postneonatal deaths	Number of infants ≥ 28 days old	Deaths (95% CI) per 1,000 infants ≥ 28 days old	
Newfoundland	6	5,394	1.1	(0.4-2.4)
Prince Edward Island	3	1,587	1.9	(0.4-5.5)
Nova Scotia	10	9,918	1.0	(0.5-1.8)
New Brunswick	15	7,892	1.9	(1.1-3.1)
Québec	132	79,461	1.7	(1.4-2.0)
Ontario	210	132,479	1.6	(1.4-1.8)
Manitoba	39	14,584	2.7	(1.9-3.6)
Saskatchewan	37	12,782	2.9	(2.0-4.0)
Alberta	50	36,777	1.4	(1.0-1.8)
British Columbia	59	44,425	1.3	(1.0-1.7)
Yukon	2	472	4.2	(0.5-15.2)
Northwest Territories	6	1,458	4.1	(1.5-8.9)
CANADA	**569**	**347,229**	**1.6**	**(1.5-1.8)**

Source: Statistics Canada. Canadian Vital Statistics System, 1997.
CI — confidence interval.

Table E4.14 **Number of infant deaths and infant mortality rate,** *Canada (excluding Newfoundland),* * *1988-1997*

Year	Number of infant deaths	Number of live births	Deaths per 1,000 live births
1988	2,703	369,247	7.32
1989	2,794	384,823	7.26
1990	2,696	397,811	6.78
1991	2,517	395,362	6.37
1992	2,381	391,718	6.08
1993	2,396	381,964	6.27
1994	2,366	378,767	6.25
1995	2,275	372,149	6.11
1996	2,013	360,450	5.58
1997	1,899	343,171	5.53

Source: Statistics Canada. Canadian Vital Statistics System, 1988-1997.
* Newfoundland is excluded because data are not available nationally prior to 1991.

Table E4.15 **Number of infant deaths and infant mortality rate, by province/territory,** *Canada, 1997*

Province/Territory	Number of infant deaths	Number of live births	Deaths (95% CI) per 1,000 live births	
Newfoundland	28	5,416	5.2	(3.4-7.5)
Prince Edward Island	7	1,591	4.4	(1.8-9.0)
Nova Scotia	44	9,952	4.4	(3.2-5.9)
New Brunswick	45	7,922	5.7	(4.1-7.6)
Québec	443	79,772	5.6	(5.0-6.1)
Ontario	728	132,997	5.5	(5.1-5.9)
Manitoba	110	14,655	7.5	(6.2-9.0)
Saskatchewan	114	12,859	8.9	(7.3-10.6)
Alberta	178	36,905	4.8	(4.1-5.6)
British Columbia	210	44,576	4.7	(4.1-5.4)
Yukon	4	474	8.4	(2.3-21.5)
Northwest Territories	16	1,468	10.9	(6.2-17.6)
CANADA	**1,927**	**348,587**	**5.5**	**(5.3-5.8)**

Source: Statistics Canada. Canadian Vital Statistics System, 1997.

CI — confidence interval.

Table E4.16 **Infant mortality rate,* by gestational age,** *Canada (excluding Ontario),** 1994-1996*

Gestational age (weeks)	Number of infant deaths	Number of live births	Deaths (95% CI) per 1,000 live births	
< 22	292	298	979.9	(956.7-992.6)
22-23	474	518	915.1	(887.6-937.6)
24-25	437	869	502.9	(469.1-536.6)
26-27	241	1,085	222.1	(197.7-248.0)
28-31	333	4,314	77.2	(69.4-85.6)
32-33	172	5,530	31.1	(26.7-36.0)
34-36	439	35,511	12.4	(11.2-13.6)
37-41	1,635	628,056	2.6	(2.5-2.7)
≥ 42	51	17,492	2.9	(2.2-3.8)
Unknown gestational age	18	2,389	7.5	(4.5-11.9)
Unlinked	64	—	—	—
All gestational ages	4,156	696,062	6.0	(5.8-6.2)

Source: Statistics Canada. Canadian Vital Statistics System, 1994-1996.

* In the birth-infant death linked file, all live births at < 22 weeks and < 500 grams were assumed to have died on the first day of life and were classified as such.

** Ontario is excluded due to data quality concerns.

Table E4.17 | **Infant mortality rate,* by birth weight,**
Canada (excluding Ontario),** 1994-1996

Birth weight (grams)	Number of infant deaths	Number of live births	Deaths (95% CI) per 1,000 live births	
< 500	495	530	934.0	(909.4-953.6)
500-749	654	1,073	609.5	(579.6-638.8)
750-999	282	1,255	224.7	(201.9-248.8)
1,000-1,249	167	1,527	109.4	(94.1-126.1)
1,250-1,499	138	1,913	72.1	(60.9-84.7)
1,500-1,999	292	7,429	39.3	(35.0-44.0)
2,000-2,499	344	25,553	13.5	(12.1-15.0)
2,500-3,999	1,498	570,021	2.6	(2.5-2.8)
≥ 4,000	160	84,738	1.9	(1.6-2.2)
Unknown birth weight	62	2,023	30.6	(23.6-39.1)
Unlinked	64	—	—	—
All birth weights	4,156	696,062	6.0	(5.8-6.2)

Source: Statistics Canada. Canadian Vital Statistics System, 1994-1996.

* In the birth-infant death linked file, all live births at < 22 weeks and < 500 grams were assumed to have died on the first day of life and were classified as such.

** Ontario is excluded due to data quality concerns.

Table E4.18 | **Number of infant deaths,* by gestational age and province/territory,**
Canada (excluding Ontario),** 1992-1996

Gestational age (weeks)	NFLD	PEI	NS	NB	QUE	MAN	SASK	ALTA	BC	YUK	NWT
< 22	14	4	21	9	133	41	20	107	82	1	0
22-23	23	6	32	14	256	67	55	161	149	3	6
24-25	29	1	39	28	242	45	69	131	136	0	2
26-27	20	3	25	14	139	38	41	67	73	0	9
28-31	28	8	25	13	198	38	48	94	87	0	7
32-33	18	2	11	12	119	19	28	70	50	0	5
34-36	29	2	33	40	253	67	49	134	136	1	12
37-41	73	21	121	120	962	233	255	554	562	11	58
≥ 42	4	0	11	5	26	15	9	19	19	0	0
Unknown gestational age	0	0	0	0	31	0	0	1	9	0	0
Unlinked	5	0	2	1	41	2	11	0	47	0	6
All gestational ages	243	47	320	256	2,400	565	585	1,338	1,350	16	105

Source: Statistics Canada. Canadian Vital Statistics System, 1992-1996.

* In the birth-infant death linked file, all live births at < 22 weeks and < 500 grams were assumed to have died on the first day of life and were classified as such.

**Ontario is excluded due to data quality concerns.

Table E4.19 Number of live births,* by gestational age and province/territory,
*Canada (excluding Ontario),** 1992-1996*

Gestational age (weeks)	NFLD	PEI	NS	NB	QUE	MAN	SASK	ALTA	BC	YUK	NWT
< 22	15	4	21	9	134	41	22	109	87	1	0
22-23	25	6	36	18	287	68	60	176	157	3	6
24-25	51	8	69	44	470	89	98	277	251	1	8
26-27	59	13	97	59	662	157	117	307	372	5	23
28-31	265	51	356	274	2,520	520	408	1,264	1,374	16	88
32-33	305	55	467	337	3,430	661	539	1,652	1,829	19	78
34-36	1,499	362	2,979	2,185	23,475	4,243	3,310	9,944	10,489	115	510
37-41	28,295	8,057	47,795	39,372	405,872	71,359	63,001	179,835	208,271	2,084	7,003
≥ 42	766	210	3,979	1,850	8,093	4,194	2,544	5,304	8,543	147	135
Unknown gestational age	10	4	50	6	6,867	19	1	1	592	2	16
All gestational ages	31,290	8,770	55,849	44,154	451,810	81,351	70,100	198,869	231,965	2,393	7,867

Source: Statistics Canada. Canadian Vital Statistics System, 1992-1996.

* In the birth-infant death linked file, all live births at < 22 weeks and < 500 grams were assumed to have died on the first day of life and were classified as such.

** Ontario is excluded due to data quality concerns.

Table E4.20 Infant mortality rate,* by gestational age and province/territory,
*Canada (excluding Ontario),** 1992-1996*

Gestational age (weeks)	NFLD	PEI	NS	NB	QUE
< 22	933.3 (680.5-998.3)	1,000.0 (397.6-1,000.0)	1,000.0 (838.9-1,000.0)	1,000.0 (663.7-1,000.0)	992.5 (959.1-999.8)
22-23	920.0 (739.7-990.2)	1,000.0 (540.7-1,000.0)	888.9 (739.4-968.9)	777.8 (523.6-935.9)	892.0 (850.2-925.4)
24-25	568.6 (422.5-706.5)	125.0 (3.2-526.5)	565.2 (440.4-684.2)	636.4 (477.7-775.9)	514.9 (468.7-560.9)
26-27	339.0 (220.8-473.9)	230.8 (50.4-538.1)	257.7 (174.2-356.5)	237.3 (136.2-366.0)	210.0 (179.5-243.0)
28-31	105.7 (71.4-149.1)	156.9 (70.2-285.9)	70.2 (46.0-101.9)	47.4 (25.5-79.8)	78.6 (68.4-89.8)
32-33	59.0 (35.3-91.7)	36.4 (4.4-125.3)	23.6 (11.8-41.8)	35.6 (18.5-61.4)	34.7 (28.8-41.4)
34-36	19.3 (13.0-27.7)	5.5 (0.7-19.8)	11.1 (7.6-15.5)	18.3 (13.1-24.8)	10.8 (9.5-12.2)
37-41	2.6 (2.0-3.2)	2.6 (1.6-4.0)	2.5 (2.1-3.0)	3.0 (2.5-3.6)	2.4 (2.2-2.5)
≥ 42	5.2 (1.4-13.3)	0.0 (0.0-17.4)	2.8 (1.4-4.9)	2.7 (0.9-6.3)	3.2 (2.1-4.7)
Unknown gestational age	0.0 (0.0-308.5)	0.0 (0.0-602.4)	0.0 (0.0-71.1)	0.0 (0.0-459.3)	4.5 (3.1-6.4)
All gestational ages	7.8 (6.8-8.8)	5.4 (3.9-7.1)	5.7 (5.1-6.4)	5.8 (5.1-6.6)	5.3 (5.1-5.5)

Gestational age (weeks)	MAN	SASK	ALTA	BC	YUK	NWT
< 22	1,000.0 (914.0-1,000.0)	909.1 (708.4-988.8)	981.7 (935.3-997.8)	942.5 (871.0-981.1)	1,000.0 (25.0-1000.0)	—
22-23	985.3 (920.8-999.6)	916.7 (816.1-972.4)	914.8 (863.3-951.5)	949.0 (902.1-977.7)	1,000.0 (292.4-1,000.0)	1,000.0 (540.7-1,000.0)
24-25	505.6 (397.5-613.3)	704.1 (603.4-792.1)	472.9 (412.9-533.5)	541.8 (478.0-604.6)	0.0 (0.0-975.0)	250.0 (31.9-650.9)
26-27	242.0 (177.3-316.7)	350.4 (264.5-444.1)	218.2 (173.3-268.7)	196.2 (157.1-240.3)	0.0 (0.0-521.8)	391.3 (197.1-614.6)
28-31	73.1 (52.2-98.9)	117.6 (88.0-152.9)	74.4 (60.5-90.2)	63.3 (51.0-77.5)	0.0 (0.0-205.9)	79.5 (32.6-157.0)
32-33	28.7 (17.4-44.5)	51.9 (34.8-74.2)	42.4 (33.2-53.2)	27.3 (20.4-35.9)	0.0 (0.0-176.5)	64.1 (21.1-143.3)
34-36	15.8 (12.3-20.0)	14.8 (11.0-19.5)	13.5 (11.3-15.9)	13.0 (10.9-15.3)	8.7 (0.2-47.5)	23.5 (12.2-40.7)
37-41	3.3 (2.9-3.7)	4.0 (3.6-4.6)	3.1 (2.8-3.3)	2.7 (2.5-2.9)	5.3 (2.6-9.4)	8.3 (6.3-10.7)
≥ 42	3.6 (2.0-5.9)	3.5 (1.6-6.7)	3.6 (2.2-5.6)	2.2 (1.3-3.5)	0.0 (0.0-24.8)	0.0 (0.0-27.0)
Unknown gestational age	0.0 (0.0-176.5)	0.0 (0.0-975.0)	1,000.0 (25.0-1.000.0)	15.2 (7.0-28.7)	0.0 (0.0-841.9)	0.0 (0.0-205.9)
All gestational ages	6.9 (6.4-7.5)	8.3 (7.7-9.0)	6.7 (6.4-7.1)	5.8 (5.5-6.1)	6.7 (3.8-10.8)	13.3 (10.9-16.1)

Source: Statistics Canada. Canadian Vital Statistics System, 1992-1996.

* Deaths (95% CI) per 1,000 live births. In the birth-infant death linked file, all live births at < 22 weeks and < 500 grams were assumed to have died on the first day of life and were classified as such.

** Ontario is excluded due to data quality concerns.

Table E4.21 **Number of infant deaths,* by birth weight and province/territory,**

*Canada (excluding Ontario),** 1992-1996*

Birth weight (grams)	NFLD	PEI	NS	NB	QUE	MAN	SASK	ALTA	BC	YUK	NWT
< 500	19	3	54	21	229	90	47	175	126	3	1
500-749	49	8	43	24	375	69	82	221	219	1	10
750-999	23	2	26	19	173	32	49	70	70	0	3
1,000-1,249	9	2	14	14	102	30	25	51	55	0	4
1,250-1,499	10	3	7	12	79	14	24	48	31	0	2
1,500-1,999	19	5	25	20	166	26	43	87	97	0	8
2,000-2,499	22	1	18	24	225	41	48	112	107	1	11
2,500-3,999	70	20	120	110	872	229	223	522	517	11	53
≥ 4,000	13	3	9	11	77	31	33	51	50	0	6
Unknown birth weight	4	0	2	0	61	1	0	1	31	0	1
Unlinked	5	0	2	1	41	2	11	0	47	0	6
All birth weights	243	47	320	256	2,400	565	585	1,338	1,350	16	105

Source: Statistics Canada. Canadian Vital Statistics System, 1992-1996.

* In the birth-infant death linked file, all live births at < 22 weeks and < 500 grams were assumed to have died on the first day of life and were classified as such.

** Ontario is excluded due to data quality concerns.

Table E4.22 **Number of live births,* by birth weight and province/territory,**

*Canada (excluding Ontario),** 1992-1996*

Birth weight (grams)	NFLD	PEI	NS	NB	QUE	MAN	SASK	ALTA	BC	YUK	NWT
< 500	21	3	54	23	249	103	48	185	135	3	1
500-749	65	14	74	45	617	132	117	352	336	4	16
750-999	68	13	129	80	757	159	130	351	331	2	14
1,000-1,249	87	19	140	106	954	200	155	417	474	5	27
1,250-1,499	107	20	135	145	1,179	232	187	533	616	9	29
1,500-1,999	378	86	637	448	4,825	838	706	2,134	2,242	25	116
2,000-2,499	1,097	287	1,993	1,520	17,546	2,669	2,288	7,624	7,658	81	289
2,500-3,999	24,562	6,880	44,382	35,191	376,367	65,006	56,773	164,397	188,105	1,889	6,257
≥ 4,000	4,890	1,432	8,252	6,595	46,118	12,005	9,688	22,874	31,440	374	1,100
Unknown birth weight	15	16	53	1	3,198	7	8	2	628	1	18
All birth weights	31,290	8,770	55,849	44,154	451,810	81,351	70,100	198,869	231,965	2,393	7,867

Source: Statistics Canada. Canadian Vital Statistics System, 1992-1996.

* In the birth-infant death linked file, all live births at < 22 weeks and < 500 grams were assumed to have died on the first day of life and were classified as such.

** Ontario is excluded due to data quality concerns.

Canadian Perinatal Health Report, 2000

Table E4.23 **Infant mortality rate,*by birth weight and province/territory,**
Canada (excluding Ontario),** 1992-1996

Birth weight (grams)	NFLD	PEI	NS	NB	QUE
< 500	904.8 (696.2-988.3)	1,000.0 (292.4-1,000.0)	1,000.0 (934.0-1,000.0)	913.0 (719.6-989.3)	919.7 (878.7-950.2)
500-749	753.8 (631.3-852.3)	571.4 (288.6-823.4)	581.1 (460.6-694.9)	533.3 (378.7-683.4)	607.8 (568.0-646.5)
750-999	338.2 (227.9-463.2)	153.8 (19.2-454.5)	201.6 (136.1-281.2)	237.5 (149.5-345.8)	228.5 (199.1-260.1)
1,000-1,249	103.4 (48.4-187.3)	105.3 (13.0-331.4)	100.0 (55.8-162.1)	132.1 (74.1-211.7)	106.9 (88.0-128.3)
1,250-1,499	93.5 (45.7-165.2)	150.0 (32.1-378.9)	51.9 (21.1-103.9)	82.8 (43.5-140.1)	67.0 (53.4-82.8)
1,500-1,999	50.3 (30.5-77.4)	58.1 (19.1-130.5)	39.2 (25.6-57.4)	44.6 (27.5-68.1)	34.4 (29.4-39.9)
2,000-2,499	20.1 (12.6-30.2)	3.5 (0.1-19.3)	9.0 (5.4-14.2)	15.8 (10.1-23.4)	12.8 (11.2-14.6)
2,500-3,999	2.8 (2.2-3.6)	2.9 (1.8-4.5)	2.7 (2.2-3.2)	3.1 (2.6-3.8)	2.3 (2.2-2.5)
≥ 4,000	2.7 (1.4-4.5)	2.1 (0.4-6.1)	1.1 (0.5-2.1)	1.7 (0.8-3.0)	1.7 (1.3-2.1)
Unknown birth weight	266.7 (77.9-551.0)	0.0 (0.0-205.9)	37.7 (4.6-129.8)	0.0 (0.0-975.0)	19.1 (14.6-24.4)
All birth weights	7.8 (6.8-8.8)	5.4 (3.9-7.1)	5.7 (5.1-6.4)	5.8 (5.1-6.6)	5.3 (5.1-5.5)

Birth weight (grams)	MAN	SASK	ALTA	BC	YUK	NWT
< 500	873.8 (793.8-931.1)	979.2 (889.3-999.5)	945.9 (902.8-973.8)	933.3 (877.2-969.1)	1,000.0 (292.4-1,000.0)	1,000.0 (25.0-1,000.0)
500-749	522.7 (434.1-610.3)	700.9 (609.3-782.0)	627.8 (575.0-678.5)	651.8 (598.2-702.7)	250.0 (6.3-805.9)	625.0 (354.3-848.0)
750-999	201.3 (141.9-272.1)	376.9 (293.5-466.1)	199.4 (158.9-245.1)	211.5 (168.7-259.5)	0.0 (0.0-841.9)	214.3 (46.6-508.0)
1,000-1,249	150.0 (103.5-207.2)	161.3 (107.2-228.8)	122.3 (92.4-157.7)	116.0 (88.6-148.3)	0.0 (0.0-521.8)	148.1 (41.9-337.3)
1,250-1,499	60.3 (33.4-99.2)	128.3 (84.0-184.9)	90.1 (67.1-117.6)	50.3 (34.4-70.7)	0.0 (0.0-336.3)	69.0 (8.5-227.7)
1,500-1,999	31.0 (20.4-45.1)	60.9 (44.4-81.2)	40.8 (32.8-50.0)	43.3 (35.2-52.5)	0.0 (0.0-137.2)	69.0 (30.2-131.4)
2,000-2,499	15.4 (11.0-20.8)	21.0 (15.5-27.7)	14.7 (12.1-17.6)	14.0 (11.5-16.9)	12.3 (0.3-66.9)	38.1 (19.2-67.1)
2,500-3,999	3.5 (3.1-4.0)	3.9 (3.4-4.5)	3.2 (2.9-3.5)	2.7 (2.5-3.0)	5.8 (2.9-10.4)	8.5 (6.4-11.1)
≥ 4,000	2.6 (1.8-3.7)	3.4 (2.3-4.8)	2.2 (1.7-2.9)	1.6 (1.2-2.1)	0.0 (0.0-9.8)	5.5 (2.0-11.8)
Unknown birth weight	142.9 (3.6-578.7)	0.0 (0.0-369.4)	500.0 (12.6-987.4)	49.4 (33.8-69.3)	0.0 (0.0-975.0)	55.6 (1.4-272.9)
All birth weights	6.9 (6.4-7.5)	8.3 (7.7-9.0)	6.7 (6.4-7.1)	5.8 (5.5-6.1)	6.7 (3.8-10.8)	13.3 (10.9-16.1)

Source: Statistics Canada. Canadian Vital Statistics System, 1992-1996.

* Deaths (95% CI) per 1,000 live births. In the birth-infant death linked file, all live births at < 22 weeks and < 500 grams were assumed to have died on the first day of life and were classified as such.

** Ontario is excluded due to data quality concerns.

Table E4.24 | **Number of cases* and rate of respiratory distress syndrome (RDS),**

Canada (excluding Québec, Nova Scotia and Manitoba),** 1989-1990 to 1997-1998

Year	Number of RDS cases	Number of hospital live births	Cases per 1,000 hospital live births
1989-1990	4,153	268,171	15.5
1990-1991	4,300	277,138	15.5
1991-1992	4,123	276,748	14.9
1992-1993	3,976	291,162	13.7
1993-1994	2,897	267,563	10.8
1994-1995	2,972	267,790	11.1
1995-1996	2,684	263,484	10.2
1996-1997	2,794	254,737	11.0
1997-1998	2,645	246,708	10.7

Source: Canadian Institute for Health Information. Discharge Abstract Database, 1989-1990 to 1997-1998.

* RDS cases include infants diagnosed during the birth admission only.

** Québec data are not included in the DAD. Nova Scotia and Manitoba are excluded because complete data for all years are not available in the DAD.

Table E4.25 | **Number of cases* and rate of respiratory distress syndrome (RDS), by province/territory,** *Canada (excluding Québec),** 1997-1998*

Province/Territory	Number of RDS cases	Number of hospital live births	Cases (95% CI) per 1,000 hospital live births	
Newfoundland	55	5,339	10.3	(7.8-13.4)
Prince Edward Island	29	1,493	19.4	(13.1-27.8)
Nova Scotia	103	9,900	10.4	(8.5-12.6)
New Brunswick	78	8,050	9.7	(7.7-12.1)
Ontario	1,481	137,173	10.8	(10.3-11.4)
Manitoba	202	14,145	14.3	(12.4-16.4)
Saskatchewan	139	12,496	11.1	(9.4-13.1)
Alberta	477	36,679	13.0	(11.9-14.2)
British Columbia	381	43,877	8.7	(7.8-9.6)
Yukon	2	432	4.6	(0.6-16.6)
Northwest Territories	3	1,169	2.6	(0.5-7.5)
CANADA*	**2,950**	**270,753**	**10.9**	**(10.5-11.3)**

Sources: Canadian Institute for Health Information. Discharge Abstract Database, 1997-1998.
Manitoba Health, Epidemiology Unit. Perinatal Surveillance Database, 1997-1998.

* RDS cases include infants diagnosed during the birth admission only.

** Québec data are not included in the DAD.

CI — confidence interval.

Table E4.26 | **Number and rate of multiple births,**
Canada (excluding Newfoundland),* 1988-1997

Year	Number of multiple births	Total births	Multiple births per 100 total births
1988	7,793	371,519	2.06
1989	8,207	387,278	2.09
1990	8,492	400,206	2.08
1991	8,147	397,611	2.02
1992	8,345	394,201	2.08
1993	8,170	384,266	2.08
1994	8,746	381,031	2.25
1995	8,682	374,476	2.28
1996	8,810	362,551	2.40
1997	8,760	345,282	2.50

Source: Statistics Canada. Canadian Vital Statistics System, 1988-1997.

* Newfoundland is excluded because data are not available nationally prior to 1991.

Table E4.27 | **Number and rate of multiple births, by province/territory,**
Canada, 1997

Province/Territory	Number of multiple births	Total births	Multiple births (95% CI) per 100 total births	
Newfoundland	127	5,447	2.3	(1.9-2.8)
Prince Edward Island	32	1,597	2.0	(1.4-2.8)
Nova Scotia	237	10,020	2.4	(2.1-2.7)
New Brunswick	196	7,969	2.5	(2.1-2.8)
Québec	1,894	80,117	2.4	(2.3-2.5)
Ontario	3,583	133,876	2.7	(2.6-2.8)
Manitoba	348	14,755	2.4	(2.1-2.6)
Saskatchewan	350	12,919	2.7	(2.4-3.0)
Alberta	968	37,154	2.6	(2.4-2.8)
British Columbia	1,091	44,913	2.4	(2.3-2.6)
Yukon	21	481	4.4	(2.7-6.6)
Northwest Territories	40	1,481	2.7	(1.9-3.7)
CANADA	**8,887**	**350,729**	**2.5**	**(2.5-2.6)**

Source: Statistics Canada. Canadian Vital Statistics System, 1997.

CI — confidence interval.

| Table E4.28 | **Number of cases and rate of neural tube defects (NTD),** *Canada (excluding Québec and Nova Scotia),* 1989-1997* |

Year	Number of NTD cases	Total births	Cases (95% CI) per 10,000 total births	
1989	329	284,590	11.6	(10.3-12.9)
1990	339	294,140	11.5	(10.3-12.8)
1991	321	293,538	10.9	(9.8-12.2)
1992	309	289,722	10.7	(9.5-11.9)
1993	281	285,790	9.8	(8.7-11.0)
1994	275	286,103	9.6	(8.5-10.8)
1995	289	282,196	10.2	(9.1-11.5)
1996	204	272,777	7.5	(6.5-8.6)
1997	197	262,741	7.5	(6.5-8.6)

Source: Health Canada. Canadian Congenital Anomalies Surveillance System, 1989-1997.

* Québec and Nova Scotia are excluded because data are not available for all years.

CI — confidence interval.

| Table E4.29 | **Number of cases and rate of neural tube defects (NTD), by province/territory,** *Canada (excluding Québec),* 1997* |

Province/Territory	Number of NTD cases	Total births	Cases (95% CI) per 10,000 total births	
Newfoundland	6	5,442	11.0	(4.0-24.0)
Prince Edward Island	0	1,570	0.0	(0.0-23.5)
Nova Scotia	10	10,017	10.0	(4.8-18.4)
New Brunswick	9	8,146	11.0	(5.1-21.0)
Ontario	106	137,046	7.7	(6.3-9.3)
Manitoba	17	14,755	11.5	(6.7-18.4)
Saskatchewan	11	12,465	8.8	(4.4-15.8)
Alberta	24	37,154	6.5	(4.1-9.6)
British Columbia	24	44,578	5.4	(3.5-8.0)
Yukon	0	455	0.0	(0.0-80.7)
Northwest Territories	0	1,130	0.0	(0.0-32.6)
CANADA*	**207**	**272,758**	**7.6**	**(6.6-8.7)**

Source: Health Canada. Canadian Congenital Anomalies Surveillance System, 1997.

* Québec is excluded because 1997 data were not available.

CI — confidence interval.

Table E4.30 **Number and rate of neonatal hospital readmissions after discharge at birth,** *Canada (excluding Québec, Nova Scotia and Manitoba),* * *1989-1990 to 1997-1998*

Year	Number of readmitted newborns	Number of live hospital births	Readmitted newborns per 100 live hospital births
1989-1990	7,518	268,171	2.8
1990-1991	8,101	277,138	2.9
1991-1992	8,231	276,748	3.0
1992-1993	8,520	291,162	3.1
1993-1994	8,709	267,563	3.3
1994-1995	9,353	267,790	3.5
1995-1996	10,000	263,484	3.8
1996-1997	9,609	254,737	3.8
1997-1998	9,748	244,264**	4.0

Source: Canadian Institute for Health Information. Discharge Abstract Database, 1989-1990 to 1997-1998.

* Québec data are not included in the DAD. Nova Scotia and Manitoba are excluded because complete data for all years are not available in the DAD.

** Because the last year of available data was 1997-1998 and a 28-day follow-up period is needed to identify neonatal readmissions, live births following March 3, 1998 were excluded.

Table E4.31 **Number and rate of neonatal hospital readmissions after discharge at birth, by province/territory,** *Canada (excluding Québec and Manitoba), 1997-1998*

Province/Territory	Number of readmitted newborns	Number of live hospital births	Readmitted newborns (95% CI) per 100 live hospital births	
Newfoundland	117	5,337	2.2	(1.8-2.6)
Prince Edward Island	23	1,559	1.5	(0.9-2.2)
Nova Scotia	246	9,837	2.5	(2.2-2.8)
New Brunswick	346	8,026	4.3	(3.9-4.8)
Ontario	5,078	135,496	3.7	(3.6-3.9)
Saskatchewan	599	12,248	4.9	(4.5-5.3)
Alberta	1,822	36,212	5.0	(4.8-5.3)
British Columbia	1,668	43,820	3.8	(3.6-4.0)
Yukon	19	452	4.2	(2.5-6.5)
Northwest Territories	76	1,114	6.8	(5.4-8.5)
CANADA*	**9,994**	**254,101**	**3.9**	**(3.9-4.0)**

Source: Canadian Institute for Health Information. Discharge Abstract Database, 1997-1998.

* Québec data are not included in the DAD. Complete Manitoba data were not available. Analyses are based on March 1997-March 1998 live births.

CI — confidence interval.

Table E4.32 **Principal diagnosis for readmitted newborns,**
Canada (excluding Québec, Nova Scotia and Manitoba), 1989-1990 and 1997-1998*

Principal diagnosis	1989-1990		1997-1998	
	Number of readmitted newborns	Percent of readmitted newborns by principal diagnosis	Number of readmitted newborns	Percent of readmitted newborns by principal diagnosis
Jaundice	1,594	21.2	3,868	38.7
Feeding problems	534	7.1	809	8.1
Sepsis	165	2.2	453	4.5
Dehydration	45	0.6	245	2.5
Inadequate weight gain	128	1.7	149	1.5
Others	5,052	67.2	4,470	44.7
Total	**7,518**	**100.0**	**9,994**	**100.0**

Source: Canadian Institute for Health Information. Discharge Abstract Database, 1989-1990 and 1997-1998.

* Québec data are not included in the DAD. Nova Scotia and Manitoba are excluded because complete data for all years are not available in the DAD.

Canadian Perinatal Health Report, 2000

Appendix F

Canadian Perinatal Surveillance System Publications (as of September 2000)

Papers Published or in Press in Peer-reviewed Journals

Chen J, Fair M, Wilkins R, Cyr M. Maternal education and fetal and infant mortality in Quebec. Fetal and Infant Mortality Study Group of the Canadian Perinatal Surveillance System. Health Rep 1998; 10: 53-64.

Dzakpasu S, Joseph KS, Kramer MS, Allen AC. The Matthew Effect: infant mortality in Canada and internationally. *Pediatrics* 2000; 106: e5.

Fair M, Cyr M, Allen AC, Wen SW, Guyon G, MacDonald RC for the Fetal-Infant Mortality Study Group. An assessment of the validity of a computer system for probabilistic record linkage of birth and infant death records in Canada. *Chronic Dis Can* 2000; 21: 8-13.

Joseph KS, Allen A, Kramer MS, Cyr M, Fair M, for the Fetal-Infant Mortality Study Group of the Canadian Perinatal Surveillance System. Changes in the registration of stillbirths less than 500g in Canada, 1985-95. *Paediatr Perinat Epidemiol* 1999; 13: 278-87.

Joseph KS, Kramer MS. Canadian infant mortality: 1994 update. *Can Med Assoc J* 1997; 156: 161-3.

Joseph KS, Kramer MS. Recent trends in Canadian infant mortality rates: effect of changes in registration of live newborns weighing less than 500 grams. *Can Med Assoc J* 1996; 155: 1047-52.

Joseph KS, Kramer MS. Recent trends in infant mortality rates and proportions of low-birth-weight live births in Canada. *Can Med Assoc J* 1997; 157: 535-41.

Joseph KS, Kramer MS. Recent versus historical trends in preterm birth in Canada (Res let). *Can Med Assoc J* 1999; 161: 1409.

Joseph KS, Kramer MS, Allen AC, Cyr M, Fair M, Ohlsson A et al. for the Fetal and Infant Health Study Group of the Canadian Perinatal Surveillance System. Gestational age and birth weight-specific declines in infant mortality in Canada, 1985-94. *Paediatr Perinat Epidemiol* (in press).

Joseph KS, Kramer MS, Allen AC, Mery LS, Platt R. Implausible birth weight for gestational age. *Am J Epidemiol* (in press).

Joseph KS, Kramer MS, Marcoux S, Ohlsson A, Wen SW, Allen A et al. Determinants of preterm birth rates in Canada from 1981 through 1983 and from 1992 through 1994. *N Engl J Med* 1998; 339: 1434-9.

Kramer MS, Demissie K, Yang H, Platt RW, Sauve R, Liston R for the Fetal and Infant Health Study Group of the Canadian Perinatal Surveillance System. The contribution of mild and moderate preterm birth to infant mortality. *J Am Med Assoc* 2000; 284: 843-9.

Liu S, Wen SW. Development of record linkage of hospital discharge data for the study of neonatal readmission. *Chronic Dis Can* 1999; 20: 77-81.

Liu S, Wen SW, Demissie K, Marcoux S, Kramer MS. Maternal asthma and pregnancy outcomes: a retrospective cohort study in Quebec, Canada. *Am J Obstet Gynecol* (in press).

Liu S, Wen SW, McMillan D, Trouton K, Fowler D, McCourt C. Increased neonatal readmission rate associated with decreased length of hospital stay at birth in Canada. *Can J Public Health* 2000; 91: 46-50.

Wen SW, Demissie K, Liu S. Adverse outcomes in pregnancies of asthmatic women: results from a Canadian population. *Ann Epidemiol* (in press).

Wen SW, Kramer MS, Liu S, Dzakpasu S, Sauve R for the Fetal and Infant Health Study Group. Infant mortality by gestational age and birth weight in Canadian provinces and territories, 1990-1994 births. *Chronic Dis Can* 2000; 21: 14-22.

Wen SW, Liu S, Fowler D. Trends and variations in neonatal length of in-hospital stay in Canada. *Can J Public Health* 1998; 89: 115-9.

Wen SW, Liu S, Joseph KS, Rouleau J, Allen A. Patterns of infant mortality caused by major congenital anomalies. *Teratology* 2000; 61: 342-6.

Wen SW, Liu S, Joseph KS, Trouton K, Allen A. Regional patterns of infant mortality caused by lethal congenital anomalies. *Can J Public Health* 1999; 90: 316-9.

Wen SW, Liu S, Kramer MS, Joseph KS, Marcoux S, Levitt C et al. The impact of prenatal glucose screening on the diagnosis of gestational diabetes *Am J Epidemiol* (in press).

Wen SW, Liu S, Marcoux S, Fowler D. Trends and variations in length of hospital stay for childbirth in Canada. *Can Med Assoc J* 1998; 158: 875-80.

Wen SW, Liu S, Marcoux S, Fowler D. Uses and limitations of routine hospital admission/separation records for perinatal surveillance. *Chronic Dis Can* 1997; 18: 113-9.

Wen SW, Mery L, Kramer MS, Jimenez V, Trouton K, Herbert P et al. Attitudes of Canadian women towards birthing centre and midwife care for childbirth. *Can Med Assoc J* 1999; 161: 708-9.

Wen SW, Rouleau J, Liu S, Sibbald B. Recent trends in male reproductive tract anomaly and cancer in Canadian provinces of Ontario and Alberta. *Teratology* (in press).

Wen SW, Rouleau J, Lowry RB, Kinakin B, Anderson-Redick S, Sibbald B et al. Congenital anomalies ascertained by two record systems run in parallel in the Canadian province of Alberta. *Can J Public Health* 2000; 91: 193-6.

Abstracts Published or Presented

Joseph KS. Secular trends in the frequency and character of multiple births International Symposium 5 — Twin pregnancies — A modern epidemic and the results of the Canadian consensus. Presented to the Society of Obstetricians and Gynaecologists of Canada, Montreal, June 2000.

Liu S, Heaman M, Demissie K, Wen SW, Marcoux S, Kramer MS. Association between maternal readmission and obstetric conditions at childbirth: a case-control study. Presented at the 13th Annual Meeting of the Society for Pediatric and Perinatal Epidemiologic Research, Seattle, Washington, June 2000: B6.

Liu S, Joseph KS, Wen SW, Kramer MS, Marcoux S, Ohlsson A, Sauve R for the Fetal-Infant Mortality Study Group of the Canadian Perinatal Surveillance System. Changing patterns of fetal and infant death due to congenital anomalies in Canada. Presented at the 13th Annual Meeting of the Society for Pediatric and Perinatal Epidemiologic Research, Seattle, Washington, June 2000: A5.

Liu S, Wen SW, Demissie K, Marcoux S, Trouton K. Maternal asthma and pregnancy outcomes: a cohort study in Quebec, Canada. *Paediatr Perinat Epidemiol* 1999; 13: A17.

Liu S, Wen SW, McMillan D, Trouton K, Fowler D et al. The association between decreased length of hospital stay at birth and increased neonatal readmission rates in Canada. *Paediatr Perinat Epidemiol* 1999; 13: A18.

Turner LA, Kramer MS, Liu S, Cyr M, Fair M, Heaman M et al. Cause-specific mortality during pregnancy and the puerperium. Presented at the 56th Annual Meeting of the Society of Obstetrics and Gynecology of Canada, Montréal, Québec, June 17-21, 2000.

Wen SW. Methodological considerations in human reproductive study of toxic exposure (abstract). *Teratology* 1997; 55: 162.

Wen SW, Demissie K, Liu S. Adverse outcomes in pregnancies of asthmatic women: results from a large Canadian population. *Am J Epidemiol* 1999; 149: S24.

Published Reports

Fair M, Cyr M, Allen AC, Wen SW, Guyon G, MacDonald RC, and the Fetal-Infant Mortality Study Group of the Canadian Perinatal Surveillance System. *Validation Study for a Record Linkage of Births and Infant Deaths in Canada.* Ottawa: Statistics Canada, 1999 (Catalogue No. 84F0013-XIE).

Health Canada. *Canadian Perinatal Surveillance System Progress Report 1997-1998.* Ottawa: Minister of Public Works and Government Services Canada, 1999.

Health Canada. *Perinatal Health Indicators for Canada: A Resource Manual.* Ottawa: Minister of Public Works and Government Services Canada, 2000 (Catalogue No H49-135/2000E).

Health Canada. *Progress Report. Canadian Perinatal Surveillance System.* Ottawa: Minister of Supply and Services Canada, 1995.

141

Published Fact Sheets

Alcohol and Pregnancy	November 1998	(English and French)
Breastfeeding	November 1998	(English and French)
Induced Abortion	April 1998	(English and French)
Infant Mortality	March 1998	(English and French)
Preterm Birth	October 1999	(English and French)
Report on Maternal Mortality in Canada	April 1998	(Bilingual)
Sudden Infant Death Syndrome	September 1999	(English and French)

Appendix G

Evaluation Form

Reader Feedback

The Canadian Perinatal Surveillance System invites you to answer a few questions about the *Canadian Perinatal Health Report*. Your answers will provide feedback on the content and usefulness of this report.

Please return the completed questionnaire to:

Reproductive Health Division
Bureau of Reproductive and Child Health
Centre for Healthy Human Development
Population and Public Health Branch
Health Canada
HPB Building #7, A.L. 0701D
Tunney's Pasture
Ottawa, Ontario
K1A 0L2
Fax: (613) 941-9927

Overall Satisfaction with the Report

For each of the following questions, please place an X beside the *most appropriate* response.

1. How did you obtain your copy of the *Report*?
   ☐ It was mailed to me as part of the initial distribution.
   ☐ I obtained my copy at work.
   ☐ I accessed it through the Internet.
   ☐ I ordered my own copy.
   ☐ Other (please specify) _____ _____

2. To what extent have you read or browsed through the *Report*?
   ☐ I have browsed through the entire document.
   ☐ I have browsed through the entire document and read specific chapters.
   ☐ I have read the entire document.

3. How satisfied are you with the following aspects of the *Report*?

   a. Length

   ☐ Too short   ☐ About right   ☐ Too long

   b. Language level (readability)

   ☐ Too high   ☐ About right   ☐ Too low

   c. Clarity of technical information

   ☐ Excellent   ☐ Good   ☐ Fair   ☐ Poor

   d. Format and organization

   ☐ Excellent   ☐ Good   ☐ Fair   ☐ Poor

   e. Use of figures/graphics

   ☐ Excellent   ☐ Good   ☐ Fair   ☐ Poor

   f. Quality of discussion

   ☐ Excellent   ☐ Good   ☐ Fair   ☐ Poor

4. How can the *Report* be improved (e.g., content, format, etc.)?

   _____

   _____

   _____

   _____

   _____

   _____

   _____

   _____

   _____

   _____

Usefulness of the Report

5. One of the goals of the *Report* is to increase awareness and understanding about the *status of perinatal health in Canada and the factors that influence health*. Overall, how successful do you think it was in achieving this goal?

   ☐ Very successful   ☐ Fairly successful

   ☐ Limited success   ☐ Not successful

6. Have you used, or will you likely use, the information in the *Report* for any of the following?

☐ Policy development   ☐ Educational activities

☐ For information only   ☐ Program planning

☐ Research and/or evaluation   ☐ Briefing notes

☐ To support intersectoral collaboration   ☐ Public awareness

☐ Other (please specify) _____

7. How useful did you find each section of the *Report*? (For each, please indicate the *most appropriate* response with an X.)

	Very useful	Somewhat useful	Not useful
Introduction	☐	☐	☐
The State of Perinatal Health in Canada — An Overview and Analysis	☐	☐	☐
Section A: Determinants of Maternal, Fetal and Infant Health	☐	☐	☐
Section B: Maternal, Fetal and Infant Health Outcomes	☐	☐	☐
Appendix A: Data Sources and Methods	☐	☐	☐
Appendix B: List of Perinatal Health Indicators	☐	☐	☐
Appendix C: List of Acronyms	☐	☐	☐
Appendix D: Components of Fetal-Infant Mortality	☐	☐	☐
Appendix E: Data Tables	☐	☐	☐
Appendix F: Canadian Perinatal Surveillance System Publications	☐	☐	☐

8. What (degree of) impact do you think the *Report* has had or will have among the following groups? (Please place the appropriate number beside *each item.*)

1 = High impact (widely used)   2 = Some impact (some use)

3 = Little impact (little use)   4 = No impact (not read or used)

5 = Unsure

____ Health policy makers within government

____ Government policy makers within other sectors

____ Local or regional health authorities

____ Non-governmental (e.g., voluntary) organizations

___ Service providers (e.g., clinicians, other health professionals, social workers)

___ Academic and/or policy researchers

___ Members of the general public

___ Media

9. Do you have a copy of the companion document, *Perinatal Health Indicators for Canada: A Resource Manual*?

   ☐ Yes   ☐ No

If no, you may obtain a copy from:

Reproductive Health Division
Bureau of Reproductive and Child Health
Centre for Healthy Human Development
Population and Public Health Branch
Health Canada
HPB Bldg. #7, A.L. 0701D
Tunney's Pasture
Ottawa, Ontario
K1A 0L2

Telephone: (613) 941-2395
Fax: (613) 941-9927

This publication can also be accessed electronically via the Internet at:
http://www.hc-sc.gc.ca/hpb/lcdc/brch/reprod.html

If yes, did you find it useful?

   ☐ Yes   ☐ No

10. Do you have other comments about the *Report* or suggestions for future reports?

   _____

   _____

   _____

   _____

   _____

   _____

   _____

   _____

   _____